RESEARCH METHODOLOGY FOR

HEALTH PROFESSIONALS

AN INTERDISCIPLINARY APPROACH

POURAN D. FAGHRI, MD, MS

ASSOCIATE PROFESSOR

DEPARTMENT OF HEALTH PROMOTION AND HEALTH SCIENCES

UNIVERSITY OF CONNECTICUT, STORRS CT

Printed in the United States of America

ISBN 1-59399-047-2

XanEdu OriginalWorks
A division of ProQuest Education
300 North Zeeb Road
Ann Arbor, MI 48106
800-218-5971

Please visit our website at www.xanedu.com/originalworks

ACKNOWLEDGEMENTS

I would like to dedicate this book to the loving memory of my late parents and brother Ahmad-Reza, Ezat, and Mehrdad Najafi whom I love and miss dearly.

I would like to thank my dear children, Tanaz and Ali, for their unconditional love and support all the time. I would also like to thank my brothers, Mehran and Shahram, for their encouragement and moral support throughout this process.

Last but not least, my husband, Amir for his love, encouragement, and mentorship to make it all worthwhile.

TABLE OF CONTENTS

PART I: INTRODUCTION TO CLINICAL RESEARCH 9

CHAPTER 1   **Introduction to Research Concept 10**
Gaining Knowledge 11
Research Question 13
Research Classifications 16
Exercises 18

CHAPTER 2   **Research Process 21**
Scientific Inquiry and Interference 21
Loop of Science 22
Hypothesizing 22
Sampling 23
Design 24
Interpretation 25
Communication 25
Stages of the Research Process 25
Exercises 26

PART II: SAMPLING & EXPERIMENTAL CONTROL 28

CHAPTER 3   **Sampling and Sampling Process 29**
Population 29
Sampling Procedures 33
Guidelines for Sample Size 36
Exercises 37

CHAPTER 4   **Variables in Research 39**
Operational Definitions of Variables 40
Types of Variables 40
Manipulation of Variables 42

CHAPTER 5   **Experimental Control 45**
Confounding Variables 45
Strategies for Controlling Confounding Variables 46
Sources of Error in Interpreting Data 50

CHAPTER 6   **Design Validity 52**
Statistical Conclusion Validity 53
Internal Validity 53
Threats to Internal Validity 53
External Validity 55
Threats to External Validity 55
Exercises 56

PART III: RESEARCH DESIGN 59

CHAPTER 7   **Descriptive Research Design 60**
Research Design in General 60

Descriptive Research Design 61
Subclasses of Descriptive Research Design 61
Potential Problem in Descriptive Research Design 65
Major Methodological Tools for All Descriptive Designs 65

CHAPTER 8   Correlation Research Design 71
Limitation of Correlation Research 73
Application of Correlation Research 73
Exercises 73

CHAPTER 9   Experimental Research Design 76
Types of Experimental Design 77
True Experimental Design 77
Quasi-Experimental Design 79
Single Subject experimental Design 81
Experimental Designs to Avoid 85

CHAPTER 10   Others Designs 87
Evaluation Research 87
Epidemiological Research 89
Exercises 92

PART IV: MEASUREMENTS IN RESEARCH 95

CHAPTER 11   Principals of Measurement 96
Measurements Applications 97
Rules of Measurements 98
Levels of Measurements 98

CHAPTER 12   Reliability of Measurements 103
Measurements Characteristics 103
Types of Measurements Error 104
Estimate of Reliability 104
Correlation and Agreement 105
Types of Reliability 105

CHAPTER 13   Validity of Measurements 110
Validity and Reliability 111
Test Validity 111
Exercises 114

PART V: DATA ANALYSIS 117

CHAPTER 14   Descriptive Statistics 118
Types of Descriptive Statistics 119
Frequency Distributions 120
Measure of Central Tendency   124
Measures of Variability 125
Coefficient of Variation 127
Z-Score 127
Standard Error of the Mean 128

CHAPTER 15   **Correlation Statistics 131**
Statistical Approach for Correlation Coefficient 132
Application of Correlation 132
Partial and multiple Correlation 133
Coefficient of Determination 134
Regression Analysis 135
Exercise 136

CHAPTER 16   **Inferential Statistics 139**
Probability 140
Standard Error of Means 140
Confidence Interval 141
Hypothesis 141
Type I Error 145
Type II Error 145
Level of Significance 145
Power Analysis 146
Parametric Statistics 149
Non-Parametric Statistics 157
Exercises 159

PART VI: RESEARCH ETHICS & COMMUNICATION 163

CHAPTER 17   **Ethical Issues in Research 164**
Defining Ethics 164
Major Issues in Unethical Research 165
Ethical Responsibility of Researcher 167
Protection of Human Rights in Research 168
Historical Background 168
Codes of Ethics 168
Institutional Review Board 171
Element of Consent Form 173
Ethical Issues in Animal Research 175
Exercises 178

CHAPTER 18   **Research Proposal Writing 180**
Purposes of Research Proposal 181
Steps in Developing Research Proposal 181
Components of a Research Proposal 184
Exercise 193

CHAPTER 19   **Research Communication 195**
Format of a Report 196
Journal Article 196
Poster Presentations 200
Platform Presentations 202
Thesis Preparation 202
Critical Review of a Research Article 205
Pyramid of Research 205
Exercise 206

APPENDICES

APPENDIX I   Additional Readings 209
APPENDIX II   Glossary of Statistical Terms 213
Appendix III   Tables of Random Numbers and Sample Size 228

Preface

I wrote this text based on the modus operandi that I have used teaching the research methods course to both undergraduate and graduate students for many years. The book is written based on personal experience and with the assumption that students come to the course with diverse backgrounds in health related areas such as dietetics, nutrition, medical laboratory, exercise, physical therapy, public health, and biomedical sciences. This comprehensive, yet practical and applicable book is written in an attempt to increase student's knowledge and grasp of the research process. The book has many interdisciplinary examples of practical and clinical application of research to teach students how to conduct their own research and how to read and understand the work of others.

In my experience of many years of teaching research methodology courses, I came to realization that students come to the course with two different backgrounds. Some students have little or no exposure to research and have little interest in conducting research. Some come to the course with an understanding that they will write a master's thesis and will have to carry out a research project. The first group usually expresses their concern and trepidation regarding the conduct of research and mostly chooses to graduate without doing a thesis. However, irrespective of what path these students choose, it is very important that both groups understand how different types of research are conducted. They must also comprehend and utilize the research done by others and incorporate the knowledge gain through this process to the advancement of their health related professions. The book is written to serve the needs of both types of students.

This book also provides across-the-board and general information on research methodology and process for doctoral students and beginning researchers. However, it is recommended that for more detailed information regarding specific techniques unique to a discipline or certain types of research, students explore more specialized research books. Additional reading materials are provided at the end of the book to help students in this regard.

Organization of the book is in such a way that will allow the students to carry out a research project from the start (identifying a research question) to the end (writing a research proposal). The book also covers issues such as research ethics, communication, and research reading.

Many people including, my colleagues, students, and friends in the scientific community had influence and encouraged me to write this book. I appreciate their inspiration and the support they provided me throughout this process.

Pouran D. Faghri, MD., MS.
Associate Professor
Department of Health Promotion and Health Sciences
University of Connecticut

PART I

INTRODUCTION TO CLINICAL RESEARCH

CHAPTER (1) Research Concept
CHAPTER (2) Research Process

CHAPTER

1

INTRODUCTION TO RESEARCH

OVERALL OBJECTIVE

To begin to understand the, who, what, why, where, and how of research

GOALS

1. Define Research
2. Understand the need for research
3. Identify research components
4. Learn to define the research question
5. Delineate different types of research

RESEARCH CONCEPT

As health care professionals, we all are responsible to make contributions to the scientific validity of our practices. That means "Research"---the discovery and validation of concepts and principals on which each of our professions is based and to improve and maximize the effectiveness of our practice. Evidence-based practice and clinical research has become an imperative part of any health profession today due to the economic challenges of our health care system. Using research effectively as a tool for understanding is a skill that can be learned. To become skillful in research one needs to understand the concepts and principals of their health related line of work. The most important concepts and principals are those related to measurements and to the scope and limitations of different research designs. A model of most effective clinical practice is one that looks at what we know now and what we need to know in order to substantiate what we do as clinicians.

Because of the importance of research in clinical practice, all the health professions now days require health professionals to gain certain fundamental skills in understanding research and interpreting research studies. Health professionals are also encouraged to participate in research activities whenever possible, especially in quality assurance programs.

GAINING KNOWLEDGE

Before you begin, look into the ways we acquire our everyday knowledge....

How does one person arrive at his/her present knowledge? How does one know that something is right? How does one know that a given treatment will work? What are the different sources of knowledge? Knowledge can be acquired in many different ways; the following are some of the most common sources of knowledge:

Custom & Tradition

"I know it because everybody knows it"

This is also called " intuition", meaning to accept a certain truth as given; without the need for external validation. Customs and traditions are good since they provide a common ground for communication and interaction within a professional society. Customs and traditions are valuable in defining the question and offering evidence as to where answers may be found, however, it is not a suitable method for validating the answer. --Be aware that many traditions have never been evaluated or tested against other alternatives.

Authority

"This is true because [some authority] said so"

Authorities can be a good source of knowledge in certain specializations. With advances in medical and technical knowledge, there are situations that one needs the advice of an expert. As researchers we may all need the help of an authority in certain areas of specialization. Authorities typically are selected based on their success, experience, and reputation in certain areas. --Be aware that if an authority's knowledge has not been scientifically documented, uncritical reliance on that authority could jeopardize your professional responsibility.

Personal Experience/Trial-and-Error

"I try different ways to solve this problem, when I get a satisfactory answer, I stop"

This approach was one of the earliest approaches in acquiring knowledge. An individual facing a problem tries one solution and if the result is satisfactory, the solution is adapted. This approach is good only when one has no other approach to solving a problem. --Be aware that using only trail and error to solve a problem has major consequences. For example, a clinician will be satisfied with the results following his or her trial and error, without knowing whether his or her result is the ultimate result. Meanwhile, there might be a better approach and the clinician will never know. Additionally, even if the results are definitive, they will never be shared with others in the same area of interest. Therefore, others might perform unnecessary trial and error of their own. Finally, trial and errors is not efficient time wise and economically.

Deductive Reasoning

This means accepting a general proposition and drawing subsequent conclusions from it. Deductive reasoning is based on *Syllogism*, which include a *Major Premise, Minor Premise,* and a *Conclusion*:
Example:
All mammals have lungs (Major Premise)
A Human being is a mammal (Minor Premise)
Human beings have lungs (Conclusion)
Sometimes, people may use deductive reasoning to gain new knowledge. --Be aware, that if the major premise is wrong all the statements that follow will be wrong.

Inductive Reasoning

This is the opposite of deductive reasoning. Inductive reasoning is a major part of the scientific inquiry, in which you generalize from a specific observation to a larger population. One chooses a sample, makes an observation and based on the results obtained from the sample generalizes to the entire population of that sample. Be aware that if the sample is not a good representation of the general population or if all the possible conditions are not observed the conclusion will be wrong.

Scientific Inquiry

This is the best approach to solving a problem. It integrates components of inductive and deductive reasoning in an orderly and organized fashion in order to analyze a phenomenon under investigation. Scientific inquiry is based on two assumptions: 1) There is an order and regulation in the events that happen in the nature, therefore they are predictable, 2) events do not occur by chance and there are reasons for their happenings.

SCIENTIFIC INQUIRY: RESEARCH APPROACH

Definition:

"Systematic, empirical, controlled, and critical examination of hypothetical propositions about the association among natural phenomena"
"Kerlinger, 1973"

Scientific inquiry requires that research proceed with:
➤ A logical order and discipline: **Systematic**
➤ Documentation of pertinent data through direct observation: **Empirical**
➤ Controlling the factors that are not directly related to the variable/s under investigation: **Controlled**

> Investigation and evaluation of other scientists' observations, examinations, and subject findings: ***Critical examination***

Therefore, research is a planned effort to obtain facts, to search for the truth, to identify and understand processes, meanings of feelings, values, behaviors, activities, and their relationships. The researcher is a person who tries to find solutions to the problems and answers to the questions in a rational, orderly, and systematic approach.

DEFINITIONS

RESEARCH

**Planned effort to:
Obtain facts
Search for the truth,
Identify and understand processes**

RESEARCHER

**Person who tries to find answer to:
Problems in a rational, orderly, and systematic approach**

RESEARCH QUESTION

Any type of research starts with a need to know the answer to a specific clinical problem. Therefore, the first step in clinical research and scientific inquiry is to identify the issues that are important to one's practice. Find out what critical questions need to be answered. Many important questions start with: What? How? When? Who? Who would be affected? What works in this specific situation? How does something work? The person may arrive at these questions simply by intellectual curiosity, or may need an answer to clinical problems. Research questions are asked for numerous reasons, all of which serve to improve, enhance, and contribute to the overall health of society.

Examples of reasons to ask a research question include:
1. to improve care
2. to prove the worth of an intervention
3. to choose the best treatment option
4. to contribute to the profession

5. Others?

Characteristics of a research question:

A research question must:
1- Be complete, correct, and well formulated
2- Be clearly spelled out
3- Lead to conclusions within the limits of the experimental design and the available data
4- Be posed in a way which is answerable
5- Use well defined terms, preferably those that have been used by others.

Defining the Research Question

In order to formulate a research question one must have the knowledge and skills to be able to find an answer to that question. This means that the person must be able to see the importance of the questions, hypothesize reasonable answers, and be able to apply research techniques to answer the questions. There are thousands of questions in each discipline. Some questions are not worth the time, effort, and money to answer them. Some questions are so complex that they are un-answerable, at least in the immediate future. Some questions are un-answerable because either the technology does not exist, or the researcher does not have the expertise to answer them. Therefore, in formalizing a research question one must consider the following:

1- Do methods exist or can they be developed?
Researchers are sometimes limited by methods available to them and make advances in the research proportionate to developing better measures and techniques.

2- Can necessary data be collected?
As a researcher you need to know whether you can collect the necessary data? Is the study feasible? For example, if your research involves human subjects participation, sometimes they may not respond in the way you projected (time wise, response wise, tolerance, acceptability of testing procedures, etc.). Pilot testing a small sample can ensure that measures, as they are proposed, can be collected.

3- Will your proposed data analysis answer the question?
Researchers should plan and make an outline of their data analysis procedures well in advance of starting to collect their data. They have to make sure that the data analysis can *REALLY* answer the question.

4- Who will use the research result?
You must decide who will use the information that you are gathering. Can it be presented in an understandable format in lay language for the general population, or can it be presented in a scientific format for a very specialized scientific group?

5- Is the question asked in a research format?
For a question to be researchable it has to be presented in a research format and must meet several characteristics; the question must be important, relevant, measurable, and ethical. Practical research methodology, materials, financial resources, time, and subjects must be available. When a question is asked in a research format, it can be answered in the best possible way. The question posed in a research format will consider the population under the study, the methodology, data collection, and data analysis plan.

Example: Does weight-bearing activities three times per week improve bone density in the elderly? (Population= elderly; methodology= cause and effect or experimental; data collection= bone density in specific intervals; data analysis= parametric statistics).

Types of Research Questions

The research question may be asked in many different ways depending on how much is known regarding the problem under study.

Descriptive Question. If you know almost nothing about the situation, you ask a descriptive research question. What is the situation? A descriptive research question tries to describe or interpret conditions or relationships that already exist and gather information about existing phenomena at a specific point in time.

Example: How do we provide dietary interventions to diabetics with limited literacy skills?

Normative Question. The researcher is making a comparison between an experiential observation and what he or she thinks the expected outcome should be. By doing this, a researcher tries to describe typical or normal values of that specific outcome. In other words the researcher is trying to establish the "norm" or the "average". The general question is: What should the situation be?

Example: What would be the typical sequence of events in the recovery process of stroke patients from the time of onset up to two years following the stroke?

Cause and Effect Question. These types of questions are used for future decision-making processes, by establishing a cause and effect relationship and establishing predictions. The general questions are: Are particular observations caused by certain factors? or Can the response of one variable be predicted by another?

Example: Does a diet high in fiber lower the blood cholesterol? Do weight-bearing activities three times per week improve bone density in elderly?

Correlational Research Question. These questions establish the relationship among 2 or more variables at a time. The purpose is to explore linear relationships between variables (to what extent are the two variables associated with each other). The general question is: Does an increase in variable A cause an increase or decrease in variable B or does it remain the same?

Example: What is the relationship between college students' GPA and their SAT?

RESEARCH CLASSIFICATION

The research process describes approaches for gathering, analyzing, and interpreting data to answer a question. Different diagrams have been used to classify research strategies according to their purposes and objectives.

Research Classification by Application

Pure, Fundamental, or Basic Research. This type of research aims to discover new knowledge without interest for its utility. It is usually motivated by intellectual curiosity and interest of a researcher in a specific problem area. The results of this research may have no practical application. In the long-term, the results of basic research may lead to practical applications, such as developing a treatment for cancer.
Example: A researcher who studies the mechanism of electrolyte transport within a muscle cell membrane is not interested in the clinical application of his or her research. He or she is doing this research for his or her own intellectual curiosity; however, the results of this research may be used for future development of a drug to treat muscle soreness (in an applied clinical research).

Applied Research. Applied research is used to solve an immediate problem without the concern for the basics of why the solution works. The idea is to improve products and processes and to test theoretical concepts. The results of this research are intended for universal population application. Clinical research is mostly applied research. An applied research may be initiated using the results of a basic research as explained above.
Example: A researcher, who evaluates the clinical effects of electrically induced muscle contractions in people with muscle paralysis, is doing an applied research. This researcher is not interested in how the electricity works at the muscle cell membrane (basic research), but how in general; this intervention is an effective way of inducing movement in people with muscle paralysis.

Action Research. Action research is similar to applied research. The interest is localized, not universal. It is also called "on the job" research. Most of the in-service training skills that are used to increase employee's knowledge in a specific area is considered an action research.
Example: A supervisor who is evaluating a new reward structure to increase the productivity of his employees is doing an action research.

Research Classification by Outcome Measures

Quantitative Research. It is the measurement of outcomes using numerical data under controlled situations. Data may be summarized and statistically analyzed using inferences. Quantitative research could be used along the range of all research approaches.

Example: A researcher who is comparing the effectiveness of a new drug for treatment of high blood pressure versus a traditional treatment for high blood pressure. He or she may randomly assign two groups of high blood pressure individuals to either receive the new treatment or the traditional treatment and after completion of the treatment, compare the changes in the blood pressure between the groups.

Qualitative Research. Qualitative research method is the collection of subjective and descriptive information under less controlled situations. It may use open-ended questions, interviews, and observation as methodological tools to collect data. The researcher tries to understand individuals' experiences for a phenomenon under investigation.
Example: How the spouses of patients with HIV feel about their partner's disease?

Research Classification by Design

A) Non-Experimental

1. *Descriptive.* Describes systematically, accurately, and truthfully a situation or area under investigation. This type of research has many different subclasses that will be discussed later.
2. *Case and field.* This is the study of the background, status, and environmental interactions of a given social unit.
3. *Correlational/Exploratory.* Investigate the extent to which variations in one factor correspond with variations in one or more other factors. It tries to explore and observe the relationships.
4. *Causal Comparative or Ex Post Facto.* Investigate possible cause-and-effect relationships by observing some existing consequence and searching back through data for a plausible cause.

B) Experimental

Overall all types of experimental research try to establish cause and effect relationships between two or more variables under controlled conditions. The result of this type of research is normally used for decision-making in a clinical or practical situation.

1. *True Experimental.* Investigate possible cause-and-effect relationships by exposing one or more groups to one or more treatment conditions and comparing the results.

2. *Single Case Experimental Design.* It is a repeated collection of information on one or a few subjects over time during the application and/or removal of treatments. It documents a particular treatment individualized to the patient with the aim of producing significant changes in a condition. In this design,

subjects act as their own control since they are compared Before/During/After the intervention.

3. *Quasi-Experimental.* Approximate the conditions of the true experiment in a setting, which does not allow the control and/or manipulation of the variables.

4. *Action.* Develop new skills or approaches in order to solve problems or improve performance in applied settings.

* *Research designs will be discussed in detail in later chapters.*

SUMMARY

Defining an appropriate question is the **"Heart and Soul"** of a good, clear, productive research.

An appropriate question should...
➤ Be derived from a perceived or determined need
➤ Determine the type of research
➤ Guide your research process
➤ Lead to valid, and constructive conclusions

EXERCISES

1- What are the ways of acquiring knowledge? How does each add to our search for truth?
2- What are the characteristics of scientific inquiry?
3- What are the differences between the types of research questions?
4- How do we classify different research approaches?
5- What are the major assumptions in scientific inquiry?

QUESTIONS FOR DISCUSSION

1- A new graduate in your discipline asks you what are the purposes of research in your discipline and who should do it. How would you answer?

2- Assume that a nurse while going through the patients files in a hospital found out that majority of deaths following the total hip and knee surgeries were due to infections following the surgery. She traced back the patients' blood cultures and found out that all the patients had staphylococcus infections and blame the hospital instrument's sanitation as a cause. Is this experimental or non-experimental? Why?

FOR STUDENTS WHO ARE PLANNING TO DO RESEARCH:

1- Identify a general problem area in which you are interested to do research. Review the literature in this area and write five questions that may inspire you to do research.

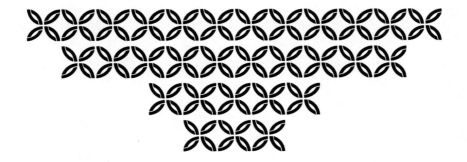

NOTES

CHAPTER

2

RESEARCH PROCESS

OVERALL OBJECTIVE

Develop an understanding of the factors that influence how to conduct a research study

GOALS

1. Understand the process for doing a sound research study
2. Understand the role of inferences in scientific inquiry
3. Demonstrate the ability to develop a research hypothesis and differentiate between different types of hypothesis
4. Distinguish between different components of research

SCIENTIFIC INQUIRY AND INFERENCES

Scientific inquiry is based on Inference. The inference is a process to generalize to a larger population based on some degree of information collected from a small sample. Information is always limited because acquiring the whole knowledge in everything is:
➤ Impractical
➤ Is not cost and time efficient
➤ If you know everything you don't have to infer
➤ Science never claims to know everything
What distinguishes scientific inquiry (research) from common sense is that scientific inquiry must follow certain *rules*.

A sound research always starts with a well thought-out *hypothesis*, identifying a *proper sample* to test the hypothesis, and developing an appropriate *design* to collect pertinent data. The next stage is **interpretation** of findings, producing new knowledge, and generating new hypotheses. The final stage is **generalization** of the results to the larger population. This process is called the **"Loop of Science"**.

THE "LOOP OF SCIENCE"

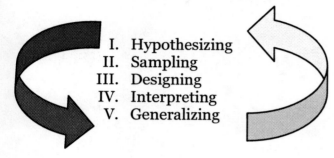

I. Hypothesizing
II. Sampling
III. Designing
IV. Interpreting
V. Generalizing

I- HYPOTHESIZING

Hypotheses are statements that predict the relationship between variables in a population. They usually incorporate phrases such as "greater than" or "less than" to indicate types of relationship. Hypotheses must be based on sound rational, and must be testable and acceptable. A hypothesis could be "deductive" or "inductive". A deductive hypothesis is based on "theoretical" premise, allowing researchers to predict outcomes under a given set of conditions. Inductive hypothesis is based on trends, regularities, patterns, or relationships that are observed in clinical practice.

In summary, a good hypothesis involves all of the above characteristics in a brief sentence and as simple as possible.

TYPES OF HYPOTHESIS

1. *No difference (null hypothesis).* There is no relationship between Variable A and Variable B.
2. *Associated difference (associative hypothesis/non directional hypothesis).* If Variable A changes, then Variable B changes, or there is a relationship between Variable A and Variable B, or Variable A affects Variable B (all examples of associated hypothesis).
3. *Directionality of difference (directional hypothesis).* If Variable A increases, then Variable B increases, or if Variable A decreases, then Variable B decreases.
4. *Magnitude of difference.* If Variable A increases by 2 points (5% or whatever), then Variable B increases by 3 points (15% or whatever).

PROCESS OF HYPOTHESIZING

The following steps must be followed to generate a sound and rational hypothesis:
1. Examine the existing knowledge base,
2. Review the relevancy of theories, and understand something of the context within which the phenomenon of interest occurs,
3. Identify problem area (choose a topic),
4. Read the theoretical research (especially the literature review sections),
5. Find a research question of interest to you (something that has puzzled previous theorists and researchers),
6. Develop appropriate hypothesis.

Research questions are longer and broader than hypotheses. Develop hypotheses that demonstrate inference by concisely reducing existing knowledge into a controllable and expressive form. Existing knowledge is what you obtain from the literature review.

More specific hypotheses are better since they will allow the researchers to use more powerful statistical analysis and do what is called affirmative or experimental research rather than exploratory or descriptive research. Experimental research is topics that have been investigated by others thoroughly and plenty of information is available for the researcher to base his or her hypothesis. Exploratory research is when the researcher knows almost nothing about the topic under investigation. Remember that you can always drop to a less rigorous hypothesis, but you cannot move up to a more rigorous hypothesis when you have already started your research.

II- SAMPLING

A sample is what one draws on to test hypotheses and to generalize based on probability theory, and frequencies. It combines inductive and deductive reasoning. In other words, sampling is the selection of the observable to make predictions about the unobservable. It considers estimates of fit between a sample (observable) and the wider population (unobservable). It should be noted that, the types of questions asked or relationships predicted will, in part, help determine the sampling plan. <u>Representativeness</u> is the most important requirement for a sample.

A *"good"* sample should present all the characteristics and differences of the population in the same proportion, as they exist in the population. A small representative sample is much better than a non-representative large sample.

Process of Sampling

The research question determines the sampling procedures. It is therefore, very important to ask a specific question and use a sampling procedure that is appropriate for that specific question. Choose a sampling procedure that has the least bias, best represents the population under study, and is practical.

Sampling procedures are discussed in detail in later chapters.

III- DESIGN

Designs are techniques and concepts that make research organized, objective, reliable, and contain operational definitions.
Designs are--
➢ Organized (relationships are stated)
➢ Objective/reliable (design can be repeated by others)
➢ Operationally defined (terms and relationships are clear)

Types of Designs
Depending on the type of research question asked, there are different types of research designs that can be used. The most basic ones are as follows:

1. *Descriptive Research Design.* The basic question is:
"What are the existing characteristics of the specific situation in the real world relative to the specific question?"
2. *Correlational Research Design.* The basic question is:
"What is the likelihood that two (or more) attributes or characteristics occur together?"
3. *Predictive Research Design.* The basic question is:
"Is there a difference between intervention A and intervention B? If there is a difference what is the magnitude of difference?"

Each design category has its own subsections that will be discussed in later chapters.

PROCESS OF DESIGNING

Choosing an appropriate design is a major step in doing research. It depends upon the knowledge, expertise and creativity of the researcher. It also depends on the type of questions asked and relationships predicted. If somebody is predicting cause and effect relationships or correlation between two or more variables, then an experimental or correlational design is appropriate. There is always a trade off between a sensible design and one that provides the highest level of confidence. Some designs might be the best designs in providing the best possible answer with the highest level of confidence; however, they may not be ethically appropriate.   In clinical research ethical issues involving human or animal subjects must be considered while choosing an appropriate design for a study.

Design with confidence: Make sure with confidence that your prospective design is most likely to be respected by the rest of the scientific community. A good design should be able to be repeated by others. The procedures must be written clearly so that if somebody else not related to the study, wants to repeat the study, they can repeat the experiment and probably get the same results. In fact, replication of a design shows the quality of the research.

IV- INTERPRETATION

Interpreting research is the most important part of the scientific inquiry. Interpretations are based on inductive reasoning, in which conclusions are drawn from the data collected from a small selected group called sample to a larger group called population. During this process, the researcher analyses the data using mathematical procedures called statistics. Statistics are mathematical tools or formulas that one can use to test whether a hypothesis is true or false. During this process the researcher makes certain assumptions about how well the sample represents the population. These assumptions are based on probability and sampling error.

V- GENERAIZEABILITY AND COMMUNICATION

The main reason for performing an interpretation is to be able to generalize. This means that conclusions are drawn based on the successful testing of all hypotheses. During generalization, the researcher must be cautious of over-generalizing to wider populations. A researcher may go beyond the sample studied, but not beyond the population that sample represents. The most important point to remember is to be cautious and reasonable in presenting your conclusions. With generalizations you are also communicating your result with others in the scientific community. You may generate more hypotheses or make recommendations for future studies based on the results of your study.

STAGES OF THE RESEARCH DEVELOPMENT

Stage I: Identify the Research Question/State your hypothesis
Stage II: Choose a sample
Stage III: Design the Study
Stage IV: Propose Data Collection Methods and Analyze the Collected Data
Stage V: Communicate the Results with Others, Generate New research Questions

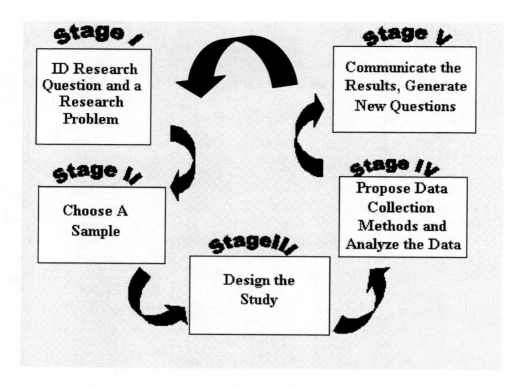

EXERCISES

1. What does an experimental approach to gain knowledge mean?
2. How do you define the term hypothesis?
3. How do we define the "loop of science"?
4. Why is generalization important in research?
5. What is the most important component of the research process that defines, the hypothesis, sampling process, and the design?

QUESTIONS FOR DISCUSSION

1. Have you ever made a decision just by your everyday observations and later realize that you were wrong?
2. What do you think about the conflicting research reports on different scientific issues that you hear on everyday news and media reports? What should you believe?

FOR STUDENTS WHO ARE PLANNING TO DO RESEARCH

1- Prioritize and list your 5 research questions (from previous section) based on the importance and interest to you? Explain why you categorized them the way you did.
2- Have you made any observation in any of the research areas under the question? If yes describe your observation.

NOTES

PART II

SAMPLING
&
EXPERIMENTAL
CONTROL

CHAPTER (3) Sampling and Sampling Process
CHAPTER (4) Variables in Research
CHAPTER (5) Experimental Control
CHAPTER (6) Design Validity

CHAPTER

3

SAMPLING AND SAMPLING PROCESS

OVERALL OBJECTIVE

Develop an understanding of how to identify a population and choose a sample.

GOALS

1. Identify procedures for defining and selecting a research sample
2. Identify different types of populations
3. Distinguish between the different types of sampling procedures

POPULATION

An important goal of clinical research is to make *generalizations* beyond the individuals studied to others with similar characteristics. The larger group from which results are generalized is called "***population***". A population under study is not restricted to human subjects. Members of an obviously distinct set of subjects, objects, events, or behaviors that meet a specified set of criteria and is the focus of an investigation is called a population. Measuring whole populations is called a "census" and is often impractical and impossible. The scope of the population to which research results will be generalized must be defined. This means that, the researcher must specify exact *inclusion* (characteristics required of the subject) *and exclusion criteria* (characteristics that prohibit participation of a subject in the study) that define a population's characteristics. Based on these criteria, a representative sample will be chosen.

TYPES OF POPULATIONS

Target Population. The target population is also called Reference Population, and is the larger population to which data may be generalized. The target population for a study of physical functioning of stroke patients is all the patients with stroke in the world. However, it is not possible to gain access to every person with stroke in the world, so you may choose your sample from a more accessible population.

Accessible Population. This is also called Experimental Population and refers to the population that you have access to and can select your sample from. It is very important that the accessible population represent the target population as closely as possible. The accessible population for a study on physical functioning of stroke patients might include all the stroke patients who participate in the outpatient rehabilitation clinics of a city.

SAMPLE SELECTION

Once the population to be studied is identified, a *representative* sample from this population must be drawn. The followings are some terms that you need to know:

"Subjects" Individual persons/animals/objects/events measured in a study.

"Sampling" Process of selecting subjects from a population; choosing a subgroup of the population so that the sample is representative of that population.

"Sample" All observations of a variable actually measured. All subjects from a population for a study, or a subset of the population

"Inclusion Criteria" Inclusion criteria describe the primary attributes of the target and accessible population. These are the criteria that would qualify someone or something as a subject. It is a set standard on what you would like to see in your subjects in order to have a representative sample. Depending on the type of question and the importance of the characteristics, you decide what the inclusion criteria will be. The inclusion criteria might be on physical, demographical, geographical characteristics, or it might be some specific health concerns.
For example: In the study on the evaluation of changes in the physical functioning of stroke patients following an intervention, the researcher may want to evaluate only those patients with hemorrhagic stroke and do not want to include other types of strokes. Therefore, the inclusion criteria would be only those with hemorrhagic stroke.

"Exclusion Criteria" Exclusion criteria describe factors that would inhibit a subject from participating in a study. These are the factors that may confound the results of the study and interfere with findings of the study. Again, depending

on the type of research question, exclusion criteria might be physical, demographical, or geographical characteristics or they may be health issues.

For example: on the above study, the researcher may exclude those stroke patients who were physically active prior to their stroke, assuming that these subjects may perform better in their physical function test, which is not necessarily due to the intervention.

A Model for Selection of Study Sample

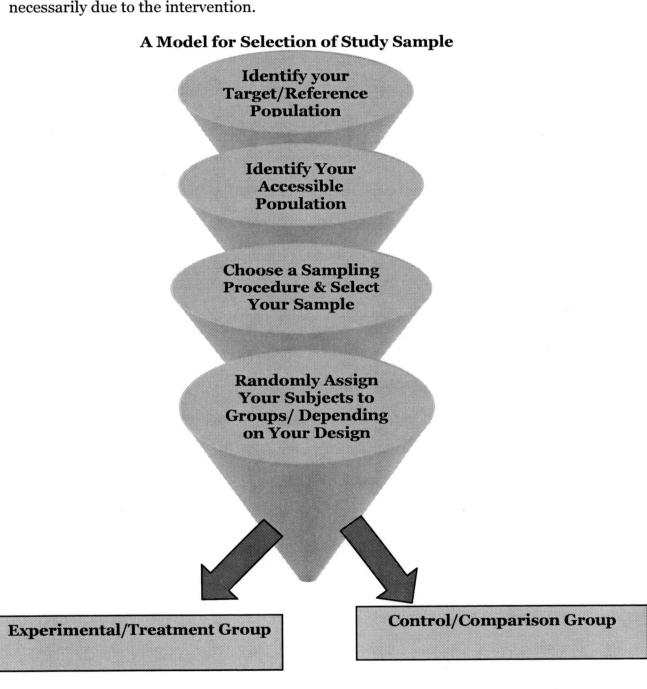

Random Selection and Random Assignment. You should not confuse random selection with random assignment. Random selection is how you draw the sample. Random assignment is how you assign people in your sample to different groups (experimental, control, etc.). People, places, events, or things are randomly selected from the accessible population, and then they will be randomly assigned to groups. In both situations each member has an equal chance of being selected to the sample and being assigned to a group. If you cannot randomly select your sample you should at least try to randomly assign them to their groups.

SAMPLING

What distinguishes clinical research from other clinical activities is making generalizations beyond the sample studied. To make an accurate generalization, the researcher must be confident that his or her sample is representative of the larger population that he or she is generalizing to. Therefore a *"good"* sample should present all the characteristics and differences of the population in the same proportion, as they exist in the population. For example: If 60% of the population is Hispanic American, then 60% of the sample should consist of Hispanic Americans. It should be noted that size is *NOT* as important as representativeness, for example: A representative sample of 50 is preferable to an unrepresentative sample of 1000.

Before assembling your sample, it is important to learn as much as possible about your population. The least amount of information you should know about your population is some of the demographic characteristics such as; age, sex, race, etc. Compiling this information regarding your population will help you with your decision regarding sample size and sampling procedure. The more diverse your population, the larger your sample size should be. Understanding the scope of variability in your population will also help you with your decision regarding data analysis and statistical power needed later.

"Sampling Error" The mean data collected on a specific variable in a sample is always different than the mean data of the target population. The difference between sample average (statistics) and population average (parameter) is called sampling error. The smaller the sampling error, the more representative a sample would be.

"Sampling Bias" Sampling bias occurs when the selected sample "over" or "under" represents the population's attributes related to the study. Sampling bias can be <u>conscious</u> (selected purposely) or <u>unconscious</u> (choosing subjects who are more cooperative, or look better) for the study. For example, in the question above the researcher may consciously only choose stroke patients who are more functional in order to show treatment effectiveness. This is considered <u>Conscious Bias</u>. In another example, a researcher may want to interview people randomly regarding a public issue. The researcher may unconsciously, only approach people who seem more cooperative, dress better, or are a specific gender or age group. This is considered <u>Unconscious Bias.</u>

SAMPLING PROCEDURES

There are different types of sampling procedures that a researcher can choose from. The research question determines the sampling procedures. A researcher must ask a specific question and use a sampling procedure that is appropriate for that question. The sampling procedure used must have the least bias, must best represent the population, and must be practical.

There are two basic approaches to sampling: **probability** and **non-probability** sampling. If you plan to draw conclusion based on your sample and generalize to the larger population, then you must use probability sampling. However, if you were only interested to see what a small group of subjects (could be representative) are doing under a certain condition or intervention, just for the purpose of illustration or explanation of a phenomenon, then you would use non-probability sampling. The most important characteristic of probability sampling is randomization (each person, object, event, etc, have the same chance of being selected).

PROBABILITY SAMPLING

Probability sampling is based on randomization. Randomization is the selection process where every subject has an equal chance of being selected and/or assigned to a group or treatment. There are different variations of probability sampling that one can use including:

Simple Random Sampling
This is a sampling procedure, when every element in a population has equal chance of being selected (random sample is unbiased). This is one of the most unbiased types of sampling. A random sample is drawn from the accessible population. The drawing of the sample could be done by using the *Table of Random Numbers* (see appendix II), using random numbers in a book, computer statistical packages, flip of a coin, drawing straws, or picking numbers from a hat, etc. The most important issue is that the accessible population must be representative of the target population. *For example*, if a researcher wants to study occupational therapists, he or she may use the directory of registered occupational therapists in the state and use that list as his or her accessible population and randomly choose a sample from this group. However, the researcher must make sure that this directory is a good representation of all the occupational therapists in the United States.

Systematic Sampling
Simple random sampling could be laborious, especially when the list of accessible population is long. In these situations the researcher may choose *Systematic Sampling*. To do this sampling, the researcher first numbers all of the members of the accessible population from one to whatever the entire accessible population is. He or she then divides the total number of people in the accessible

population to the number of samples needed. Therefore, to select a sample of 200 from a list of 2000, the researcher divides 2000 by 200 and the result is 10. This is called the *Sampling Interval*. The researcher then chooses the first number to be drawn from the accessible population using the table of random samples, and then adds this number to the sampling interval until the entire sample is chosen. For the above example, assume that the first number chosen from the accessible population using the table is 23. Therefore the first person to be chosen is number 23, next is number 33 (23+10), next is number 43 (33+10), next is number 53 (43+10) and so on... This is less laborious since as soon as you find the sampling interval and randomly select the first number from the accessible population the rest is easy.

Stratified Random Sampling

In simple or systematic random sampling the distribution of characteristics of the sample may be different from the population just by chance. For example, from a list of occupational therapists by chance all the numbers drawn might be male. This may not be a representative sample of the population of occupational therapists. Stratified random sampling is a sampling method that corrects for the bias/error that is part of being a member of a certain group. The researcher selects a "stratum" that he/she wants to be represented in proportion to the total, and then selects randomly from strata, e.g., males-females, age groups, etc. In the example of occupational therapist, the researcher may want to have an equal number of males and females in her sample in order to have a good representation of gender. She can identify the two strata of "male" and "female" and randomly select 100 males and 100 females for her study. This is called proportional stratified sampling, since we are assuming that our accessible population consisted of an equal proportion of males and females. Please note that, stratification increases the precision of estimate only when the stratification variable is closely related to the variable of experimental interest. If the gender is not an issue in regards to your question, you may not want to stratify your sample to male and female.

Disproportional Sampling

When the proportions of the population and the stratified sample are not equal, the researcher may use disproportional sampling. In the example of occupational therapists, if from the list of 2000 registered occupational therapists (accessible population), 1200 are male and 800 are female. To select a representative sample of 100 male and 100 female, each female has a 1 out of 8 (total of 100 out of 800) chance of being selected, while each male has a 1 out of 12 (total of 100 out of 1200) chance. Researchers may deal with this situation either by not paying attention and continue the random selections and leave the proportional representation to chance, or he/she may use disproportional sampling to control the situation. Disproportional sampling uses a weighing procedure in which it proportionally weights the probability that any one subject from the sample will be chosen and multiplies the final data by weights. In our example the researcher may go ahead and randomly select 100 male and 100 female from the list. However, when data are analyzed the male scores are multiplied by 12 and female scores are multiplied by 8. Therefore, in any mathematical manipulations the male scores will be larger than the female scores and proportional representations of each group are differentiated in the total data set. In this procedure, the relative contribution of these scores to the overall data is controlled while the average scores of each group are not affected.

Cluster or Multistage Sampling

This type of sampling entails consecutive random selection of a series of units within the population. This is for situations where the accessible population is too large to randomly select a sample from it. The researcher then identifies a series of units within the population and randomly selects from these units until the sampling is completed.

For example, you may want to survey the attitudes of clinical exercise physiologists regarding working with elderly. You identify your accessible population as all clinical exercise physiologists in the United States. However, it is not economical nor time efficient to randomly select from this large group size. You may use multi-stage sampling, by first randomly selecting 2 or 3 states out of 50 states. Then from each selected state randomly select two or three hospitals, and from each selected hospital randomly select 4 or 5 clinical exercise physiologists and administer your questionnaire to this group. Area probability sampling and random-digit dialing are examples of this type of sampling. The major disadvantage of cluster sampling is the probability of increased sampling error. With every sampling during different stages, there is a sampling error, increasing the inaccuracy of the final sample.

NON-PROBABILITY SAMPLING

In clinical research sometimes it is impossible to select a random sample, either due to ethical issues or a small number of eligible samples. In these situations the researcher may choose to sample through non-random selection. In non-probability sampling because not all elements of the population have a chance of being selected, the sample might not be a representative sample and data should be analyzed and generalized with caution. There are different variations of non-probability sampling that one can use including:

Convenience Sampling

This is the most common type of non-probability sampling in clinical research. The researcher selects "n" number of subjects in a "series" who meet inclusion criteria (first come first serve basis). The most common ways of doing this type of sampling is through volunteers, by posting the "wanted subject" posters. This sampling has an unknown amount of bias; since the researcher may unconsciously choose those who look better, respond better, etc. Another major limitation of this type of sampling is self-selection. Subjects may participate because they are interested in the study, may benefit from it, or for other reasons. Therefore, they are not representing the general population who may also have subjects with no interest or benefit from the study and who may respond differently. Because the sample is not a representative sample of the larger population generalizeability and external validity is questionable.

Quota Sampling

This is like convenience sampling with quotas and proportions. There might be some unknown characteristics of the population that may confound the data. The researcher uses quota sampling to control these characteristics. For example, a researcher may find that males and females respond differently to an intervention. He/she may decide to use gender as the quota and recruit 100 males and 100 females. The researcher could also use convenience sampling, however, the goal is to recruit 100 subjects for each quota, and as soon as they reach 100 for each quota he/she will stop recruiting. This sampling is also based on a first come first serve basis and has all the limitations of convenience sampling.

Purposive Sampling

The researcher might be looking for rare subjects with some specific characteristics. The researcher then hand picks subjects on the basis of specific criteria or a set of defined characteristics. For example, the researcher may go through patients' records and identify those with specific characteristics and choose them for the study. This sampling is like convenience sampling with the difference that in purposive sampling explicit choices are made to select the sample rather than simple availability. Since a researcher exercises his/her right to choose subjects, this type of sampling may have unlimited bias. For example, the researcher may identify those who meet the specific characteristics but do not choose them because they have other limitations that do not allow them to perform at the ultimate level that the researcher is looking for, therefore, he/she may eliminate them from the study.

Snowball Sampling

This type of sampling is useful when subjects with specific characteristics are hard to find. The researcher identifies a subject with the specific characteristics and asks the subject to find others with the same characteristics as themselves and introduce them to the researcher. This process of "snow balling" or "chain referral" is continued until an adequate sample is obtained. For example, a researcher may be interested in doing an investigation involving people with HIV who are also drug users, he or she may find one person with these characteristics and then ask these subjects to identify others with the same characteristics and have them contact the researcher.

GUIDELINES ON SAMPLE SIZE

Sample size is the number of subjects actually included and measured in a study. Adequate sample size should permit the study to be sensitive enough to determine a statistically significant difference, if it exists, and to be able to generalize the results. A well-selected representative sample is better than a poorly selected non-representative sample. Larger samples do not produce better results.

In research and statistics, capital (N) always refers to total sample in an accessible population, and small (n) refers to the number or subjects in the selected sample studied for the investigation.

Rules on Sample Size

1. A sample NEVER exceeds 50% of the population
2. 30 samples per group is normally the minimum acceptable size
3. Usually a larger sample generates more statistical power
4. Sample size depends upon the type of research
5. Descriptive research requires a larger sample
6. Experimental research requires a smaller sample
7. The larger the variation in the population (and sample) on the variable under study the larger the number needed in the sample.
8. Larger sample size reduces sampling errors
9. Statistical procedures such as Power Analysis can be used to determine appropriate sample size.
10. The *MOST* important element is *HOW* the sample is selected (representation)

EXERCISES

1- How do researchers decide on an appropriate sample size?
2- What is the accessible population and why is it important?
3- When should a researcher use non-probability sampling?
4- What is the major draw back to cluster sampling?
5- What is sampling bias and why should researchers avoid it?

QUESTIONS FOR DISCUSSION

1- For each of the following, determine what type of sampling has been used and why?

- o A Spanish teacher wants to select five students out 61 students in her class and send them to Spain. She writes down everybody's name on pieces of papers, then drops these papers into a hat and draws five names out of the hat.
- o A witness is asked to pick out criminals from a lineup in a prison
- o A researcher goes to a classroom and asks for volunteers
- o Selecting the first names that appear in the alphabetical order of a phone book
- o Sending a survey to the entire households in a town.
- o Dialing random telephone numbers
- o Flipping a coin while reading the names from a list.

FOR STUDENTS WHO ARE PLANNING TO DO RESEARCH

1. What type of sampling will you be doing for your study?
2. How are you going to decide about the sample size for your research?

NOTES

CHAPTER

4

VARIABLES IN RESEARCH

OVERALL OBJECTIVE

Develop an understanding of the definition of different variables in research and how they influence the conduct a research study

GOALS

1. Demonstrate the ability to identify different types of variables in research.
2. Understand the difference between conceptual definitions and operational definitions.
3. Demonstrate the ability to identify different types of variables and how to manipulate them

VARIABLES

Variables are characteristics of interest to the researcher and are considered structural elements of the research question. To perform a research study, a researcher identifies a number of variables to be studied. These variables are either investigated for their relationship with each other or are described, as they exist in nature. Variables have more than one value and can be measured either quantitatively (height, weight), or qualitatively (sex, color, or type of disability). If a characteristic has only one value, it is called a *Constant.*

In descriptive or correlational questions, variables are observed either for their relationships among each other or are described accordingly. In experimental research, the researcher observes the changes in one variable and predicts the outcome in another variable. For example, in a research study to evaluate the effect of a medication X on blood pressure, medication X and blood pressure are variables of interest to the researcher. The researcher evaluates the effect of different dosage of the medications (different values) and predicts the outcome of the blood pressure in response to those changes.

Operational Definition of Variables

Variables must be operationally defined at the start of the research. Developing *operational definitions* for every variable under investigation, is one of the important steps in a research process. It has to be done before hypothesis formulation and design process initiation. Operational definitions are definitions of the variables as they are used in research, which might be different, than dictionary or conceptual definitions. Defining these definitions are important so others can understand and replicate the research. Therefore, researchers must define their variables very precisely, especially the dependent variables.

There is a difference between **conceptual definitions** and **operational definitions**. Conceptual definitions are dictionary definitions, which may be different than operational definitions that you define for your research variables.

For example a researcher may want to measure subjects walking speed and define the speed as measuring the number of steps per minute. This *operational definition* of speed is very different than the *conceptual definition* of speed you find in the dictionary.

Types of Variables

Independent Variable/Treatment Variable (IV). This variable is also called predictor variable or treatment variable and is a factor or intervention that cause changes in another variable or outcome.

Dependant variable (DV). This variable is also called the outcome variable or the response variable and is measured following the controlled manipulation of the independent variable by the researcher who sets its "value". The researcher assumes that under controlled conditions, any change in the dependent variable is caused by or is associated with the "value" of the independent variable. It should be noted that the researcher cannot manipulate the value of the dependant variable and it depends entirely on the independent variable. However, the researcher can manipulate the values of the independent variable. In other words, the independent variable is manipulated to determine its effect on the dependent variable.

Mathematically we can presume that the dependent variable is a function of the independent variable

$y = f(x)$ (y is a function of x)

y = dependent variable

x = independent variable

Independent Variables (IV) are given "values" called <u>levels.</u> Every IV has at least 2 <u>levels.</u> You may have more than one IV in a research question but do not confuse the IV with levels of IV.

Example: 1- What would be the effect of a low fat diet on the blood cholesterol of a group of cardiac patients? IV = diet (it has two levels: a group who would receive the diet and a group who would not). DV = blood cholesterol

2 - What would be the effect of a low fat diet on the blood cholesterol of a group of cardiac patients after 3, 6, and 9 months? IVs = diet (two levels) and time (three levels: at 3, 6, and 9 months), DV = blood cholesterol

The Value for an IV Can Be Explained in Two Ways:

1- Qualitative IV. Qualitative variables deal with differences in kind and classify subjects based on their already established attribute or categories. It allows the researcher to evaluate the contrasts and deals with variability in kind or type. Values are assigned according to a classification already set in the design, so they have no meaning except being labels. Qualitative variables may only have two levels in which case they are called "Dichotomous/binomial (sex =male, female), or they may have more than one value in which case they are called "Polychotomous" (health = poor, fair, excellent).

2- Quantitative IV. Quantitative variables deal with variations in the amount, which can be measured quantitatively, such as dosage of medication, age, height, and number of treatments. Variables that are measured quantitatively, normally determine the nature or shape of a relationship.

OTHER CLASSIFICATIONS OF VARIABLES

Order/Continuous Variable. When a variable covers a range of conditions with some order, that variable is called an Order or a Continuous Variable. For example, if a researcher is interested in evaluating the effect of a treatment on subjects after 5, 10, 15 minutes of application. Time in this example is one of the IVs with four levels of 0, 5, 10, and 15 minutes (treatment is the other IV). The researcher measures the dependent variable (or response to treatment) during these time periods and observes the trend or relationship between each time period.

Active Variable. Whenever a researcher can manipulate different levels of the IV by randomly assigning the subjects to these levels, the IV is called Active Variable.
Example: What would be the heart rate response to a high, medium or low intensity aerobic exercise? In this example, the researcher randomly assigns the sample to receive one of the intensities of exercise and evaluates the subjects' heart rate responses. Exercise is an active independent variable with three levels (low, medium, and high) and heart rate is a dependent variable.

Attribute variable. Whenever, a researcher is interested in examining subjects within their natural groupings according to natural distinctiveness and does not have the power to assign subjects to levels, he is examining attribute variables.

Example: A researcher who is interested in differences between male and female in response to an intervention. The researcher cannot randomly assign subjects as male or female; they are either male or female. In this example the researcher studies subjects in their natural grouping and makes the comparison. Other examples of attribute variables are age group, occupation, or weight, etc.

MANIPULATION OF VARIABLES

When researchers intentionally perform an operation by intruding the IV to at least one group of subjects and observe the effects of an experimental condition (dependent variable) on the subjects, he/she is manipulating the independent variable.

The researcher can manipulate active variables, attribute variables or both active and attribute variables.

Manipulation of Active Variables. The researcher manipulates the levels of the IV by assigning subjects to varied conditions.

Example: What would be the effect of different doses of medication X on blood pressure? A researcher randomly assigns the subjects to three or more groups and gives them a different dosage of medication and compares different groups' blood pressure response. In this example, medication is an active variable.

Manipulation of Attribute Variables. These types of variables (age, sex, etc.) can be manipulated by the researcher, but cannot be randomly assigned to the subjects (male or female). Since subjects are examined according to predetermined natural characteristics, this approach is considered *"ex-Post-facto"*. *"Ex-Post-facto"* research allows the researcher to consider relationships; however, it does not allow the researcher to control the experiment and therefore, limits the interpretation of cause and effect.

Example: What is the difference between cerebral palsy (CP) and spinal cord injured (SCI) patients in response to muscle strengthening exercise? (IV: type of disability with two levels (CP and SCI), DV: muscle strengthening exercise). In this example type of disability cannot be randomly assigned, subjects are either CP or SCI.

Manipulation of Both Active (Assignable) and Attribute Variable. Depending on the type of research question, the researcher can manipulate both active and attribute variables. For example: How would CP and SCI subjects respond to aerobic exercise vs muscle strengthening exercises? In this example, exercise (active) is an independent variable with two levels that can be randomly assigned, and CP and SCI (attribute) can be characterized as two types of disability, which is an independent variable that cannot be randomly assigned. Therefore the researcher randomly assigns two groups of CP and two groups of SCI subjects to either receive aerobic or muscle strengthening exercises and compare the effects between groups.

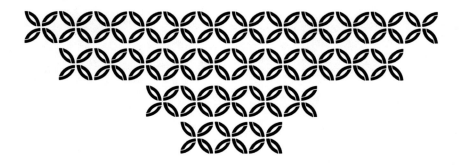

NOTES

CHAPTER

5

EXPERIMENTAL CONTROL

OVERALL OBJECTIVE

Develop an understanding of Experimental control in research

GOALS

1. Learn how to identify confounding variables in a research study
2. Identify sources of error in research
3. Define experimental control and strategies to control confounding variables

EXPERIMENTAL CONTROL

In experimental research the goal is to establish a *cause-and-effect* relationship between a specific behavior (independent variable, IV) and an observable response (dependent variable, DV). This however, must be done based on a logical structure, or design, within which the investigator systematically instigates changes (IV) and then observes the consequences of the changes (DV). During this process, the researcher is responsible for controlling all aspects of the project except the one being studied. This means that, in order for the researcher to state with confidence that the observed changes in the dependant variable are due to the manipulation performed on the independent variable, she/he must identify all relevant sources of variation (variables) that may affect the observation and develop a plan to control them.

Confounding Variables

Any variable that may affect the DV, and may confuse the interpretation of the data if not controlled are called confounding, intervening, or nuisance variables.

These are any factors not directly related to the purpose of the study, but may affect the dependent variable, if uncontrolled. They can contaminate the IV such that their separate effects are masked and the researcher cannot state with confidence that changes in the DV are due to direct manipulation of the IV.

Confounding variables can be:

1. Extrinsic Factors. These are factors that emerge from the environment and or the experimental situation. For example: subjects may respond differently to exercise in a cold or hot environment. If the researcher is only interested in subjects' response to exercise, environmental temperature may affect subjects' response. Therefore, temperature is considered a confounding factor and must be controlled by the researcher either by eliminating it or incorporating it into the design, so its effect can be evaluated during data analysis procedures.

2. Intrinsic factors. Intrinsic confounding factors are personal characteristics of the subjects of the study that may change. These are much harder to control, since they may change with each subject and each situation. For example: blood pressure fluctuates in a person from time to time. Or a subject may fatigue during a test without the knowledge of the researcher and therefore respond differently to an intervention. There are strategies that a researcher may use to control for confounding variables.

STRATEGIES TO CONTROL THE CONFOUNDING VARIABLES

To control for the effects of extraneous factors that occur within the experimental situation, the researcher must either eliminate them or provide assurance that they will affect all groups equally. Some of the strategies that may be used are as follows:
1. Random Assignment
2. Selection of control group
3. Appropriate research protocol
4. Blinding
5. Reduce inter-subject differences

1- *Random Assignment.* For this strategy, the researcher identifies the sample to be tested and then randomly assigns them to different treatment groups. Each subject has an equal chance of being assigned to either the experimental or control groups and therefore, the confounding variable/s will affect both groups irrespective of their assignments. For example, in the question above if subjects are randomly assigned to the experimental and control groups, they will be performing in both environments irrespective of their group assignments. In this case, the confounding effect of temperature will affect both groups, and any change at the completion of the study could be assumed to be due to the IV.

2- *Selection of Control Group.* One of the most practical ways to rule out extraneous variable's effects on the IV is to randomly assign subjects to control and experimental groups. The control group will not receive the intervention and will be observed in their normal setting while; the experimental group will receive the intervention. It is assumed that confounding variables will affect both groups and therefore any changes in the experimental group will be the result of the intervention.

3- *Research Protocol.* Research protocols are an important part of a research study. They are written like a recipe book for all to follow. Using an accurate and concise protocol, the researcher first identifies the confounding variables and controls them by either eliminating them (which sometimes is not possible) or provides guarantee that they will affect all groups equally. Below are some of the steps used to develop a concise research protocol.

I. Identify which factor will mostly contaminate the dependent variable
II. Develop a consistent protocol
III. Develop clear criteria for assigning the independent variable
IV. Train those who collect the data and test them for their reliability
V. Control subjects' activities that directly effect the data collection
VI. Reduce the potential for observational bias

4- *Blinding Procedures.* Observational bias is one of the most important concerns in experimental research. Although random assignment may control for this situation, subjects' knowledge of the type of intervention that they are receiving or investigators' knowledge of subjects' assignment may play a role in their responses to the intervention. The purpose of blinding procedures is to overcome these concerns. The most complete blind design involves hiding the identity of group assignments from the subjects, those who provide treatment, those who measure outcome variables, and those who reduce and analyze the data. This procedure is called **Double Blind Study**. Double blind study is hard in clinical research since sometimes the tester is part of the treatment. For example, in physical therapy, many times the researcher is interested in comparing two different treatment approaches, in which the tester is part of the treatment approaches and it will be hard to blind the tester. In these situations, the researcher may hide the group assignments from the subjects; this is considered a **Single Blind Study.** In a single blind study, only the tester knows the identity of the treatment. The researcher may use Sham or placebo.

Placebo: This is when the control group receives an irrelevant treatment. It differentiates the effects of any change from the effects of a specific change that was introduced for experimental reasons.
Example: Giving sugar pills to the control group as a placebo, when evaluating the effects of a new drug, or using teaching technique that seems different than regular teaching for the control group, when evaluating a new teaching technique.

Sham. Sham procedures are used when something false pretending to be genuine is given to the subjects. It may involve deception.

Some types of research do not require blinding for response variable. For example, historical research does not require blinding, since researchers cannot control for what happened in the past. This is considered *ex-post-facto*, however, blinding may be required during the assessment and data analysis.

5- *Reduce Inter-Subject Differences*. Sometimes personal traits or characteristics of subjects being studied may affect their response to an intervention (i.e., gender, age, weight, etc). Therefore it would be hard for the researcher to know whether the response to an intervention is a real response or due to those personal traits. The following are some of the design strategies that a researcher may use to reduce inter-subject variability.

➤ "Selection of homogeneous subjects." Choosing subjects who have the same characteristics of the extraneous variable. For example, if men respond differently than women to an intervention, only choose men or women for testing. The major problem in this approach is that generalization (to the larger population) will be limited (can only be generalized to male or female) and therefore the application of the results will be limited.

➤ "Blocking." In this strategy the researcher builds extraneous attribute variables into a design by using them as independent variables, creating blocks of subjects that are homogeneous for the different levels of the variable. Each category is called a ***block*** and the variable is called a ***blocking variable***. When subjects in each block are randomly assigned to treatment groups, the design is called ***randomized block design***. This procedure could be used to control the confounding effect of an attribute variable (i.e., gender, age, level of education, etc.). It allows the researcher to systematically manipulate them by building them into the experimental design as an independent variable.

Example: Males and females may respond differently to an exercise program, therefore, sex could be used as a blocking attribute variable with two levels (male and female). The researcher chooses one male group and one female group and then randomly assigns subjects in each group to an experimental (exercise) and a control group (non-exercise).

➤ "Matching." In this procedure, subjects are matched based on specific characteristics or attribute. It is done, by identifying subjects with the same characteristics and then randomly assigning them to groups. Matching could be done on one or more characteristics. The more the characteristics the harder the selection of subjects and assignment will be. When only two groups are involved, the technique is called **match pair design.** When subjects are matched on the basis of pre-score measurement on the dependent variable the technique is called ***Rank order design.***

Example: If we are concerned with the effect of subjects' height on our dependant variable. The matching procedure could be used to guarantee an equivalent group of tall and short people (make sure you operationally define the short and tall in your procedures) in the experimental and control group. This approach is a **match pair design** since only one variable (height) is used as a matching variable. Two subjects from each block (two tall or two short) are matched as closely as possible and then randomly assigned to experimental or control group. This will allow the same number of tall and short people in both control and experimental groups. Therefore, if there are any differences due to height it will affect both groups the same way.

➤ "Using Subjects as Own Control." It exposes a subject to different levels of independent variable and compare the response within the same subject. When all the subjects are exposed to all levels of independent variable, the independent variable is called **repeated measure or repeated factor**. The design used for this approach is called **repeated measure design**. Subjects are used as their own control; therefore, all the subjects' characteristics are the same for all levels of experiment. This approach is not appropriate when carryover effects are likely, since previous exposure may affect the subject's response to the next level of independent variable.

Counterbalance: To control for carry over effect or learning effects, one of the strategies is to do counterbalance. This is a common form of manipulation to gain control in a research study. The design requires that all subjects receive all treatments but in different orders. The testing should be far enough to reduce fatigue, learning, etc, effects and close enough to allow fair comparison between each treatment.

Example: If a researcher is interested to know the effect of body position (supine or prone position) in CP patients' performance during an exercise intervention. A group of CP patients will be tested once during supine position and once during prone position and their responses will be compared. The IV in this example is position with two levels (prone and supine) and is considered a repeated factor. In this example subjects are used as their own control. To control for carryover effect, the decision as to which treatment a subject will receive first will be determined randomly.

➤ "Statistical Techniques." These techniques are applied when other manipulations are not possible. The researcher knows, at the beginning of the study, that the experimental group differs from the control group in some variable. The statistical technique used in these situations is called Analysis of Covariance (ANCOVA). The ANCOVA techniques adjust the differences in scores among groups at the end of the study based on differences in initial scores among the groups. If there was still a difference between the control and the experimental groups after final scores were adjusted, the researcher may conclude, that the experimental treatment was effective.

Covariates are the scores that are obtained at the beginning of the study.

Variates are the scores that are obtained at the end of the study.

ANCOVA is the adjustment between differences in the covariate (initial score) and the variate (final score).

Example: If a researcher is evaluating the effect of an intervention on subjects' walking speed and realizes that the subjects in the experimental group are significantly taller than those in the control group. She/he may use AVCOVA to adjust for the differences in the walking speed between the groups at the beginning and adjust that for the final score.

SOURCES OF ERROR IN INTERPRETING DATA

Researchers must be aware of the sources of error that are the results of atypical manner of response by either the subjects or tester that may affect the dependant variable during an experiment.

1- *"Hawthorne Effect."* Subjects may perform in an atypical manner because they realize they are participating in an experiment.

2- *"Placebo Effect."* Subjects may believe treatment is supposed to change them so they respond with a change in performance.

3- *"John Henry Effect."* Control group tries to outperform the experimental group because they are considered "Secondary Citizens" (Avis effects: we are second but we try harder).

4- *"Rating Effect."* This situation occurs when the initial impression of the tester of a subject's response to a test influences his or her impression for future measurements. This is especially important for situations where the measurement is subjective and the tester is part of the measurement system. For example, if an intervention is supposed to increase muscle tone, and the researcher is measuring muscle tone using a nominal scale from 0 (no tone) to 4 (high tone). The researcher may unconsciously overrate the experimental group since the intervention is supposed to increase tone. Rating errors can be minimized by not looking at previous ratings.

5- *"Experimenter Bias Effect."* Bias of a researcher can affect the outcome of the whole study. Experimenter bias may influence methodology, treatment, and data collection. Bias usually favors the experimental group. Experimenter bias may be controlled by single or double blind approach.

6- *"Subject-Researcher Interaction Effect."* Subjects may respond differently to a certain type of researcher (female/male, older/younger).

7- *"Post Hoc Error."* This form of error assumes a cause-and-effect relationship when there is none.

NOTES

CHAPTER

6

DESIGN VALIDITY

OVERALL OBJECTIVE

Understand design validity and its importance in research

GOALS

1. Understand the concepts of internal and external validities
2. Identify threats to internal and external validity
3. Develop strategies to control the threats to internal and external validities

DESIGN VALIDITY

The goal of experimental design is to establish a cause-and-effect relationship between the independent (IV) and the dependant variables (DV). There are three main design validities that must be established for an experiment to be valid.

Statistical Conclusion Validity: Statistically establishes the cause-and-effect relationship between independent and dependant variables.

Internal Validity: Establishes that IV causes change in the DV, by controlling all the confounding variables.

External validity: Generalizes the results from a small sample to the larger population with the same characteristics by establishing that the sample is a good representation of the larger population it represents.

Statistical Conclusion Validity

For an experiment to be valid, the statistics used to analyze the data must be appropriate for that study. It should not violate assumptions for statistical tests and must have enough power to prove relationships if it exists. The analysis must have high reliability and validity with the lowest error rate and must be appropriate for the proposed study design. For example, a researcher cannot use inferential statistics for descriptive research, or correlational research and try to establish a cause and effect relationship, when it does not exist.

Internal Validity

A design is said to have internal validity, when the researcher can say with confidence that the changes in the dependent variable are due to manipulations performed by the researcher on the independent variable. Confounding/extraneous variables may affect the dependant variable, and the changes in the DV may be due to these nuisance variables. Internal validity is the degree to which an experiment discards other possible explanations of the results. A true research experiment eliminates all aspects, other than the independent variable, that can influence changes in the dependent variable. True experiments have a high degree of internal validity; because of the significant level of control imposed by a researcher, such as performing randomization and using a control group.

Threats to Internal Validity

Threats to internal validity refers to the potential for confounding factors to interfere with relationship between the IV and DV and include:

"History."
These are events other than the intervention that could influence the results during the course of a study. The history effect could happen only on long-term studies (changes in the law, education). For example, a researcher may be interested in an educational intervention that would increase the use of car seats for young children, during the intervention a law may passes that requires everyone to use car seats for their children. In this situation, there will be an increase in car seat use (DV), but this increase may not be due to the educational intervention (IV).

"Maturation"
These are changes over time resulting from processes within a subject (i.e., aging, natural progression of a disease). These changes may cause a subject to respond differently on second measurement of the DV, which may not be related to the IV (i.e., growing older, getting worse, etc). Maturation is a common threat in longitudinal studies that require long-term involvement and repeated measurements of a DV on the subjects.

"Repeat Testing"
In situations where subjects are repeatedly tested under the same condition, changes may occur in the DV, due to repeated testing. Subjects may become

more comfortable, familiar, and smarter when performing the test, therefore, score differently. These changes in DV are due to a learning effect not manipulation of IV.

"Instrumentation"

Instruments play a major role in establishing the internal validity in an experiment. Changes in the calibration of instruments or changes in the way a tester records data for a specific behavior could produce different results in the DV. Sometimes, an observer becomes more experienced and skilled at performing measurements between a pretest and posttest, so the difference in the DV is not due to the intervention but due to the observer's experience.

"Attrition"

In any research that deals with human subjects, there is always the possibility that subjects will drop out of the study before the study is completed. This is also called experimental mortality. A researcher does his/her best to have control and experimental groups that are comparable in their characteristics that are important to the study. If during the study, a majority of the subjects in either the experimental or control group drops out, the sample is no longer representative of the larger population. There is also the possibility of not establishing a cause-and-effect relationship simply due to a lower number of subjects. To control for this problem, researchers should predict the possibility of subject attrition and recruit more subjects for the study. There are also statistical procedures that may be used to accommodate for these situations.

"Statistical Regression"

Statistical regression deals with reliability of the instrument or test. If an instrument is not reliable, it can produce different results for the same measurement. Therefore, there is always a tendency for extreme scores to move toward the average after repeated testing. This is called **regression toward the mean**. Usually after a few testing, the very high scores reduce to the lower scores and very low scores increases to the higher scores, while the middle scores remain unchanged. Since sometimes subject selection in research is based on a subject's score on a specific test, statistical regression may cause a major dilemma in subjects' selection. For example, a researcher may be interested on those students who get a grade of B or above on their exams. If during the period of subject selection, the teacher gives extremely hard exams or extremely easy exams, students may get scores that are not representative of their true grades.

It is recommended that if specific instruments are used for tests, the researcher should calibrate the instruments regularly and if possible use the same instrument for all measurements. Also, if a response variable naturally fluctuates, try to get more than one measurement and use the average as the final score. For example, if the response variable is blood pressure and the researcher knows that there are fluctuations on the subjects' blood pressure from time to time, he or she may measure each subject's blood pressure three times and report the average of these three measurements each time.

"Selection/Sampling Bias"
Selection/Sampling biases refer to differences between groups due to a selection process. For example choosing more responsive, more cooperative subjects for the experimental group. Random assignment could control for this bias.

"Diffusion of Treatment"
Sometimes during a study the experimental and control groups may communicate with each other and the control group may perform the same types of activities that the experimental group is doing without the knowledge of the researcher. At the completion of the study there might be no differences between the groups not necessarily because the intervention was not effective, but because both groups received the same intervention. This is considered diffusion of the treatment.

"Floor/Ceiling Effects"
Floor/Ceiling effects occur when a researcher is trying to measure a nonexistent, a very high, or low-level behavior, or trying to improve an already outstanding performance or behavior. She/he may see no change, because it cannot get any better or be measured by the instrument.

"Selection Interaction"
Some of the threats to internal validity may interact with selection, which may produce changes on the dependant variable that may look like the effect of independent variable. Selection interaction occurs when factors leading to selection interact with maturation, history, or testing. In selection interaction with maturation, one of the groups (experimental or control) may mature at different rates. For example, if you are evaluating changes in the motor skills of children and you are comparing 5 years olds with 15 years olds they mature at different rates and cannot be compared. Selection interaction with history happens when groups are coming from different settings with different history. Finally selection interaction with testing or instruments occurs when two different instruments with different levels or intervals of measurements are used to measure a response. For example, measuring subjects' height in centimeters and inches.

External Validity
External validity is the degree to which results can be generalized to the larger population that is outside of the experimental situation. External validity deals with sample selection and representation. A study has strong external validity when the sample is a good representative of the larger population.

Threats to External Validity

"Multiple Treatment Interference"
When subjects are concurrently and randomly receiving treatments other than the experimental treatment the effects of other therapies on specific performance,

or the effects of the order of treatments cannot be separated. Therefore, the researcher cannot say with confidence that the same changes will occur in the population that the sample is representing.

"Interaction Effects of Testing"
In the process of taking a test, the sample becomes different from the population it is supposed to represent, because the sample knows more, they act differently. For example, if a knowledge test is repeatedly administer to the subjects, just by taking the test repeatedly, the subject may learn more and the results of the test will be different.

"Interactive Effects of Selection Bias"
The interaction between inclusion criteria and treatment (include those who meet the inclusion criteria in the experimental group and those who don't in the control group). Random assignment controls for this condition.

"Experimental Arrangement"
Physical arrangement of testing room may affect how subjects respond to treatment. For example, testing subjects under abnormal conditions (i.e., small room, hot environment), which may not be the normal condition for the population that the results will be generalized to.

SUMMARY

All threats to internal and external validity are never totally controlled and excluded. Sometimes researchers may make trade-offs between them to get the most feasible arrangement and experimental results.

EXERCISES FOR CHAPTERS 4-6

1- What is the difference between conceptual and operational definition?
2- What is the least number of dependent variables that an experiment can have?
3- Can an experiment have more than one independent variable? If yes, give an example.
4- In an experiment, the tester is very friendly with the experimental group and encourages their participation and performance, however she is not friendly with the control group. What type of threat may affect this experiment?
5- If a researcher is studying the effect of seat belt use in reducing car accidents and during her research a law passes that makes using seat belts during driving mandatory, what type of threat is affecting this experiment?
6- Can a researcher overcome all the threats to internal and external validity? If yes, how?
7- What threat to validity deals with whether or not you can generalize the results of your study to the larger population?

QUESTIONS FOR DISCUSSION

1- Identify an experimental situation and name a variable that you can manipulate, and then identify a confounding variable that may affect your dependent variable.

2- Discuss an experiment that you may not be able to do due to ethical or legal reason.

FOR STUDENTS WHO ARE PLANNING TO DO RESEARCH

1- If you are doing an experiment, identify all the threats to internal and external validity of your experiment and explain how you will control for them.

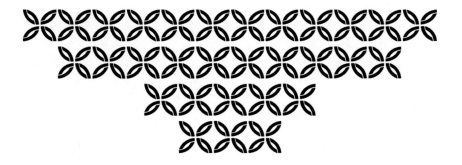

NOTES

PART III

RESEARCH DESIGN

CHAPTER (7)   Descriptive Research Design
CHAPTER (8)   Correlation Research Design
CHAPTER (9)   Experimental Research Design
CHAPTER (10) Others Designs

CHAPTER

7

DESCRIPTIVE RESEARCH DESIGN

OVERALL OBJECTIVE

To develop an understanding of the different types of descriptive research designs and how they are most appropriately used.

GOALS

1. Understand research design in general
2. Differentiate between different types of descriptive research designs
3. Describe the subclasses of descriptive research design and give an example of how each is used

RESEARCH DESIGN IN GENERAL

The main purpose of research is sequential and orderly development of a body of knowledge through several research types and designs. Research designs are techniques and concepts that make research systematic, objective, consistent, and contain operational definitions. Therefore, designs are said to be:

➢ Organized (meaning that relationships are stated)
➢ Objective, Consistent (meaning that research can be repeated by others)
➢ Operationally defined (meaning that terms and relationships are defined)

TYPES OF RESEARCH DESIGNS

A researcher could add to the body of knowledge utilizing several different types of designs. However, it is the research question that determines the research design. Usually, the general sequence of a research design if you know nothing or almost nothing about the topic proceeds from:

Descriptive → correlation → predictive

The sequence of a Descriptive Research design proceeds from:

Qualitative (nominal) form → normative form

The sequence of a Predictive Research design proceeds from:

Simple → complex

➢ *Descriptive Research Design.* The basic question is:
"What are the existing characteristics of the specific situation in the real world relative to the specific question?"
➢ *Correlational Research Design.* The basic question is:
"What is the likelihood that two (or more) attributes or characteristics occur together?"
➢ *Predictive Research Design.* The basic question is:
"Is there a difference between intervention A and intervention B? If there is a difference what is the magnitude of the difference?"

DESCRIPTIVE RESEARCH DESIGN

Purpose
The purpose of a descriptive research design is to determine the major distinctiveness of a population, as it presents in nature. The researcher looks at the aspects of a sample in a natural setting in a planned, controlled way, and records his or her observations. Descriptive research can be retrospective, e.g., if 70% of the sample has X-characteristics, then 70% of population does also. It is said that descriptive research is the foundation for building new knowledge.

Characteristics of Descriptive Research
1. Nature assigns the treatment
2. The researcher does not manipulate the variables
3. The researcher observes the characteristics of a population, as it is, in a natural setting to draw conclusions

Subclasses of Descriptive Research
a. Qualitative Research
b. Nominal Descriptive Research
c. Normative Descriptive Research
d. Historical Descriptive Research
e. Developmental Descriptive Research
f. Review of Literature
g. Meta-Analysis

a. Qualitative Descriptive Research.

A qualitative researcher studies people or situations either individually or as a group in their socio-cultural environment. The focus of this research is on people and the meanings that they are attached to or are derived from their experiences. The major emphasis is on the experience as a whole and the meaning of that experience for a specific individual or population. For example, a qualitative researcher might be interested in how a society looks at death and dying. These are life states that are ingrained in the cultural and religious values, as well as in economical and social conditions of the culture. For the researcher to explain these conditions he/she must look at the issue from a holistic and social structure view and put an emphasis on the totality of the experience and the meaning of that experience. She/he might decide to go into that culture and live the life the same way as they do to get the same feelings or experiences, or she/he might use informers to get information about the culture. The researcher may use one-on-one interviews, group discussions, or surveys to find the answer. At the end, the researcher writes a tick description of the whole issue related to the phenomenon under study for the specific culture.

The methodological approaches for qualitative research are: Philosophical Analysis, Phenomenology, Ethnography, Life History, and Ground Theory.

* Students are encouraged to read other books on qualitative research if interested in this type of research.

b. Nominal Descriptive Research (Case Study).

Nominal descriptive research, which is also called Case Study, is more appropriate when you practically know nothing about the topic under investigation and can't ask any specific questions. It is for situations where your sample is extremely small (usually one) and the population for your sample may not be clearly defined. The typical approach is to find an interesting question regarding a specific individual or situation. The researcher then plans to make some observation of that situation or individual. An important point is that the procedures for observation and how it should be done has to be planned in advance. The researcher must know exactly what he or she is looking for and how he or she is planning to record or measure those observations. The researcher then makes an in-depth description of the condition or response to the treatment and analyzes it to understand factors important to etiology, care, and outcome of that subject, group, social unit, etc. In the majority of case studies, the only tools used are direct observations and/or interviews.

Steps to Follow in a Case Study

1. Full history of subject (remember: in research a subject is not always a human subject. It could be a human, animal, object, event, institution, etc.)
2. Describe problems, symptoms, prior treatments, demographic and social factors that are relevant to subjects (i.e., patient care, prognosis)

3. Describe elements/expectations of the treatment plan
4. Document all interventions, subject's responses and complete follow-up

c. Normative Descriptive Research.

This is a natural step after nominal research and considers an expansion of nominal research. It means to make "norm", or "average/typical". It defines average or typical characteristics of a given sample. The researcher based on a few case studies or nominal descriptive research and after observing some similar cases and recording the same types of observations, draws a conclusion by making his or her results into an average or norm response for that specific population. In normative descriptive research the researcher should be able to identify this new population characteristic. For example, the researcher may identify the average age of patients who have specific characteristics, or the average range of motion or the average for any other characteristic of interest for a specific population.

d. Historical Descriptive Research.

The focus of historical research is on past events rather than present events and tries to describe what *was* instead of what *is.* A historical researcher uses document analysis as the methodological tool. Because the researcher is relying on sources that either have lived in the past or have information about the past, the validity and reliability of the source is very important. The basis of historical research is an explanation of an event recorded in original historical documents *(primary sources) or* evaluation and explanation of those documents provided by other researchers *(secondary sources).* Therefore both the *primary and secondary sources* must be valid and reliable sources.

Example: A researcher might be interested to know how the American Disability Act of 1990 came to pass. She/he will do a historical review of the past, from legislative policy, to advocacy, and specific circumstances that end up with this legislation. During the process the person may use both primary and secondary sources for information recording.

e. Developmental Descriptive Research.

This type of descriptive research, describes the temporal sequence of events/incidences/natural history of a variable over a long period of time. It uses direct observation and repeated measurements over time. Usually is difficult, time consuming, and very expensive. For example, developmental charts that most pediatricians use to evaluate the sequential physical development of children are the results of these types of research.

Subclasses of Developmental Descriptive Research

1. Cohort Study (longitudinal): For this type of research, a cohort of a sample is followed over a period of time and observed for the development of a number of characteristics. Since a sample must be followed for a long period of time (usually years), this type of research is very time consuming and expensive. The most important threats to validity of this research are testing, history, and attrition. If the subject became familiar with tests and are able to learn from them, then they may perform differently on future tests (testing), or if during the study a law is passed that may affect the subject's response, their response might change (history). There is also the possibility of losing subjects during the study (attrition). However, depending on the type of research question these threats may or may not exist.

Example: Do physical therapists' attitudes toward elderly individuals change as they grow older themselves? A cohort of recent graduates of physical therapy programs could be identified and followed for ten or twenty years and every year a questionnaire evaluating their attitude toward elderly will be given to them, the changes in their attitudes will be then recorded each year and analyzed at the end of the study.

2. Cross-Sectional Methods: In cross-sectional methods, groups of subjects who are stratified based on important characteristics are studied at one point in time. Researchers then report their findings based on the development of a number of characteristics in these subjects over time. Since data are collected at one point, this type of study is less time consuming and more efficient than a longitudinal cohort study. Testing or history do not pose a threat to the research, as all the subjects are tested once at the same time. However, selection is a major threat in this type of research. People might have different life experiences, education, and personal life styles; that is, it is difficult to know to what extent the results reflect the effect of age or the passage of time versus the effects of extraneous variables.

Example: The above question regarding the attitude of physical therapists toward elderly, as they grow older, may be answered through cross-sectional design by selecting samples of physical therapists in different age groups and evaluating their attitude toward the elderly then comparing the results between different age groups.

f. Review of Literature.

In this type of descriptive research, the researcher who is usually an expert in a given field, reads, understands, integrates, and summarizes a significant body of literature and publishes the results for others. Note that almost every published article in a professional journal has a section on review of literature, which summarizes what others have done for the issue under study. However, there is some descriptive research where the research question is: what does the literature say about a specific area of reseach? The researcher searches systematically in the library for answers and summarizes the findings in a separate review article. Remember that no new data is gathered; therefore, the review of literature by itself is not considered "research".

g. Meta-Analysis.

Meta analysis goes one step further than a review of literature and performs its own compilation and quantitative re-analysis of published data in a specific area of research. The researcher tries to establish criteria for evaluating quality, reliability, and validity of the studies in a specific problem area. In meta-analysis the researcher may analyze other researchers' data or develop his or her own data analysis plan and provide new data, therefore, meta-analysis could be considered "research".

Potential Problems in Descriptive Research

Potential problems in descriptive research are: 1) improper sampling, 2) asking the wrong question, 3) collecting data inappropriately in order to answer the question, 4) making incorrect inferences, and 5) finally unconscious bias in selecting parameters to be observed.

Due to the nature of descriptive research, the researcher may consciously or unconsciously bias the data in the direction that supports his or her hypothesis. The bias may also occur by the respondent. For example, since major methods for descriptive research are surveys and interviews, the subjects may respond to the questions in a way that they think they should be responding or in a way they think would please the researcher, which may not be their true response. Also subjects may respond differently just because they are aware that they are being observed. It may not be possible to take biases completely out of descriptive research, however, researchers must be aware of them and do their best to apply constrains whenever possible to control for these biases.

Major Methodological Tools for All Descriptive Research

I. Survey.
➤ *Questionnaire:* Self-administered
➤ *Interview:* Administer by the researcher

II. Case study.
This method of research describes a subject's behavior across time. This method was discussed in the previous section.

I. **Surveys.** This is one of the major methodological tools for collecting descriptive data. It is used primarily to measure characteristics of a population by generating a series of questions that are pointed toward a group of subjects. It is typically conducted with large samples and makes it possible to describe the population parameter and predict relationships. The survey questions may be posed through questionnaires, telephone or face-to-face interviews.

"Questionnaires"
The survey questionnaires are constructed so that they can be self administered by the respondents using pen and paper. The most common form of distribution is through the mail. Advantages of questionnaires are: 1) they can reach a large number of people with minimal expenditure, 2) numerous variables can be measured, 3) it is more time efficient since the respondents answer the questions on their own time, and 4) the researcher could use the data for multiple purposes.

The disadvantages of surveys are: 1) low response rate, which compromises the external validity (responses of 60-%-80% are excellent, 30%-60% are considered realistic), 2) time consuming, and 3) the researcher may use bias in reporting the results. The researcher does not directly observe the respondents' behavior or attitudes, but only records the respondents' report of them. In this case, there is always potential for bias or inaccuracy.

"Interviews"

Interviews may be performed face-to-face or through the telephone. An interview may be *structured or unstructured*. In *structured* interviews the researcher asks specific questions from all of the subjects and gives them all the same choice for responses. In *unstructured* interviews the researcher poses the questions informally and discusses the issues and concerns with subjects informally. The researcher then writes a tick analysis of the respondent responses. This is the major method of data collection in qualitative research.

The major disadvantages of interviews are: 1) time consumption, 2) high cost, and 3) lack of anonymity. There is also the possibility of biases both on the side of researcher and the respondent.

STEPS IN DESIGNING A SURVEY

a. Guiding Questionnaire: This process involves developing a questionnaire around a model that provides a framework for operational definitions, for choosing particular target populations, and for choosing particular variables that are most tolerant, relevant, and important to the purpose of the research.

b. Review of an Existing Instrument: The researcher should perform a comprehensive review of literature and study all the existing questionnaires pertinent to the study.

c. Preliminary Draft: Draft a preliminary questionnaire related to the study based on the information gathered in the previous steps.

d. Pilot Testing: Before administering the questionnaire to the entire sample, it is recommended that the researcher choose a small sample from the population under investigation and implement the questionnaire. He/she may also consult with experts in the field and get their input and improve the questionnaire further.

e. Additional Revisions: Additional changes could be done based on pilot testing.

f. Final Draft: Develop the final draft of the questionnaire.

g. Administration of the Survey: Administer the survey to representative sample.

TYPES OF SURVEY QUESTIONS

"Open-Ended Questions" These types of questions allow the respondents to reflect their feelings and opinions regarding the question asked, without biases or limitations enforced by the researcher.
Example: What part of your vacation was most enjoyable to you?

"Close-Ended Questions" These are like multiple-choice questions that somehow may limit the respondent's opinions or feelings. They do not allow expression of the respondent's own personal viewpoint. There is also the possibility of bias by researchers since they may only include the responses that they are interested in as part of the answer choices.

Example: Which of the following parts of your vacation did you find most enjoyable?

[ ] Relaxing at the beach
[ ] Shopping
[ ] Dinning out
[ ] Sleeping

Sometimes the researcher is interested in more than one answer to a question.

Example:
Which of the following parts of your vacation did you find most enjoyable?
                                        yes   no   unsure
[ ] Relaxing at the beach
[ ] Shopping
[ ] Dinning out
[ ] Sleeping

"Double-Barreled Questions" Assessing two things with one question ("or", "and"). These types of questions are not recommended. It is better to ask two questions and assess activities separately.

Example: How many times a week do you walk **or** ride a bicycle?

"Frequency Measure Questions" The researcher is interested in quantifying behavior in terms of time and frequency.

Example:
How often do you drink alcoholic beverages?

[ ] Every day
[ ] Once a week

[ ] Once a month
[ ] Never

Rating Scales
These are a set of numerical values assigned to responses that represent the degree to which the respondent possesses a particular attitude, value, or characteristic.

Categorical Scales. These scales are used with nominal measurements. Normally in a question, the respondents are asked to assign themselves according to several classifications. These scales are usually used for variables such as gender, level of income, level of education, race, etc. The researcher usually reports categorical scales as frequencies or percentages. For example, 70% percent of respondents were male, or 30% of respondents had a high school level education.

Summative Scales. These are scales that can create a summary score from a series of items, which together indicates characteristics that a subject may posses. Usually the scores are summed around one dimension of a characteristic and all items that are measured must only measure that characteristic. The total score with all items having the same weight and contributing an equal weight to the total then will be presented as how much of an attribute the person has (i.e., quality of life measure).

Cumulative Score. Is a type of summary score that demonstrates an accumulative characteristic, which a subject may posses. Each item represents an increasing amount of the characteristic being measured. For example, questionnaires of activities of daily living (ADL) use this type of scoring. The higher the score the more active a person is.
Example:
1. *Likert Scales.* This is a type of summative scale that is usually used to measure a characteristic, attitude, or value. A series of questions are presented to respondents. They are asked to rank their responses according to the rank presented.

For example: For each statement below, indicate whether you strongly agree (SA), agree (A), disagree (D), or strongly disagree (SD).

1. Knowledge of the new developments in exercise science is important for all exercise physiologists.
(SA), (A), (D), (SD)

2. Physical therapists must learn and understand statistics during their entry-level programs.
(SA), (A), (D), (SD)

3. Writing a thesis must be a graduation requirement for all master level students.

(SA), (A), (D), (SD)

The data will then be summarized for each item and may be given values from 0 (SD) to 3 (SA). At the end, the researcher reports the percentage of subjects that responded to each of the values.

2. *Visual Analogue Scale.* This is a simple way of assessing the intensity of a subjective experience by the respondents (i.e., pain intensity, or taste intensity). Usually a fixed line is drawn or a bar graph with a fixed length is presented to the subjects. The subjects then will be asked to place a mark along the continuum line corresponding to their perceived level of that characteristic. Usually the subjects are told that they should look at the line from the bottom to the top, the top being the highest possible intensity and the bottom being the lowest possible intensity. Researchers then develop their own measurement scales by, for example making a line at 50 cm and measuring the length of the places that the subjects marked and presenting that point as the perceived intensity (at 50cm, the highest and 0 cm, the lowest possible).

3. *Guttman Scale.* This is another kind of cumulative scale, in which a series of questions or statements are presented to the subjects that reflect increasing intensity of a characteristic or attitude. In the scale researchers must make sure that with each statement they only measure one dimension within a series of possible responses. The total score will be calculated and presented as how much of a characteristic a subject has. Tests of physical functions that are used in physical therapy are examples of this type of scale.

Example:
   1- I can get out of my house without any help
   2- I can get around my house including up and down the stairs
   3- I can walk around our neighborhood without any difficulty
   4- I have no physical condition which limit my activities
   5- ....
   6- ....

The questions could go on, the subjects will then be given the choices of agree (1) and disagree (0), the total data will then be calculated for all items and the maximum score will be equal to the number of items in the scale. Remember that with this scale you have to make sure that you are measuring only one dimension of a characteristic, then the person with a total score equal to the total number of items has the attribute and the rest could be compared accordingly.

There are many other types of scales and questionnaires available that students who are interested may use. Additional references are provided in Appendix I.

NOTES

CHAPTER
8

CORRELATION RESEARCH DESIGN

OVERALL OBJECTIVE

To develop an understanding of correlation research design and how it is most appropriately used.

GOALS

1. Define correlation research design in general
2. Understand how to interpret correlation coefficients
3. Recognize the limitations of correlation research

CORRELATION RESEARCH DESIGN

Correlation research design examines the relationships among 2 or more variables at a given time. It is based on a mathematical measure called Correlation Coefficient. It tries to explore a linear relationship between two or more variables and to what extent the variables are associated with each other. The description of the relationship between two variables explains how accurately scores in one variable could be predicted from another variable. It also explains the degree to which differences between two variables can be attributed to the same determining factor. It is very important that the two scores be paired in some way, meaning that they should be either taken from the same individual, event, situation, or be reasonably related and paired with each other. For example, a researcher might find a positive correlation between an increase in watching TV and diagnosis of skin cancer in the last decade. However, there is no logical relationship between the two variables.

Correlation Coefficient = r

This is a mathematical measure of the extent to which two or more related paired phenomena or events tend to occur together. It can range from +1 (perfect positive correlation) to −1 (perfect negative correlation).

Positive Correlation. Where you see one, you tend to see the other.
Negative Correlation. Where you see one, you tend not to see the other.

Example:
Does an increase in variable A cause an increase or decrease in variable B or does it remain the same?

Examples of r for Linear Relationships (Types):

Perfect positive correlation
(r = 1.0)

Perfect negative correlation
(r = - 1.0)

Moderately high positive correlation
(r = + 0.8)

Moderate negative correlation
(r= -0.7)

Low negative correlation
(r= ±0.6 or lower)

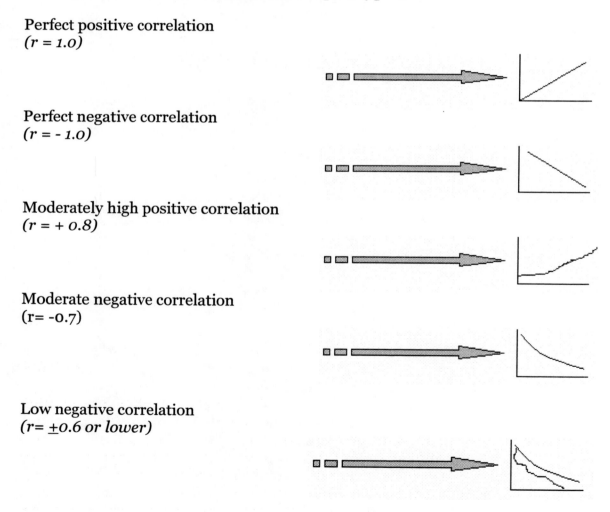

Coefficient of Determination = r² = Percentage

Correlation coefficient should not be interpreted in terms of percentages. For example, a correlation of 0.80 does not means that when one variable varies the other variable varies 80 percent of the time. For this type of information, researchers use another determination called, Coefficient of Determination, which means, when one factor varies, the other factor varies by a specific percentage of the time. Coefficient of determination is the square of the Correlation Coefficient.

Example: If r = .80, then r ² = 64%

Percentage of change in one variable in relation to another variable is 64 percent of a time. Another important factor regarding correlational research is that, when we say two variables correlate with each other, it does not mean that one is caused by the other. Correlational research does not establish cause and effect relationships. As a matter of fact two-correlated variables might be both caused by a third variable.

Limitations of Correlation Research

➤ Never infer causal relationships
➤ High r can be the result of random/systematic bias
➤ Both variables could be cause by a third extraneous variable

Application of Correlation Research

Correlational research can be used to:

➤ Establish theoretical or logical relationships between two variables
➤ Postulate a more specific experiment
➤ Establish test-retest reliability

EXERCISES FOR CHAPTERS 6-7

1- Why must a researcher have a design before starting a research study?
2- What is the general sequence of a research design if you know nothing or almost nothing about the topic?
3- If a researcher conducts a survey of college students to study their perception of college life, what type of research is she/he doing?
4- A case study involves how many subjects?
5- A researcher administers a test of intelligent to a group of young children annually to evaluate changes in intelligence over time, what type of research is she/he doing?
6- A researcher is studying the relationship between SAT scores in high school and GPA in college, what type of research is she/he doing?

7- Two researchers conducted two different correlational studies and their **r**-values were (+0.7) and (−0.7) respectively, can we say that the first study has a higher correlation than the second study? Why? Why not?

QUESTIONS FOR DISCUSSION:

1- Name a topic in your field that you want to do descriptive research on? Which type of descriptive research would be most appropriate? Why?
2- Discuss a historical research that you have heard or read about.

FOR STUDENTS WHO ARE PLANNING TO DO RESEARCH

1. If you are doing descriptive research what type will it be? What are the variables that you will be studying?
2. If you are doing correlation research, what are the variables that you are interested in evaluating their relationships?

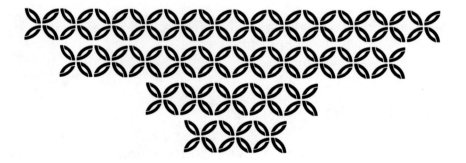

NOTES

CHAPTER

9

EXPERIMENTAL RESEARCH DESIGN

OVERALL OBJECTIVE

To develop an understanding of the experimental research design and how it is most appropriately used

GOALS

1. Develop an understanding of experimental research design and manipulation of variables
2. Differentiate between different types of experimental research designs
3. Identify experimental designs to avoid

EXPERIMENTAL RESEARCH DESIGNS

Experimental research designs provide a systematic and structural evaluation of data to establish a cause-and-effect relationship between two sets of variables; the independent, or treatment variable (IV) and the response, or dependent variable (DV). These designs are the most effective and expensive way to find an answer to a research question. There are some requirements that should be met before starting an experimental design:

1- You need to have a control group and they must be chosen randomly. This group must be statistically equal on the characteristics under investigation to a randomly assigned experimental or treatment group.

2- Both the experimental and control groups must come from the same population, and must be "*statistically equal*" at the start of the experiment based on the characteristics under investigation. This will allow you to say with confidence that any changes that occur after the intervention are due to your intervention, not by chance.

3- You may have more than one control group or more than one treatment group. The most important points are that each group should have an equal number of subjects (usually between 25-30) and must be statistically equal. It is desirable to run a pretest on the dependant variable(s) on all of the subjects to develop some baseline data and to establish equality between groups for later statistical analyses and for better documentation of the effect of the IV on the DV.

4- Every experiment must have a posttest and the findings are usually compared between the pretest and posttest and between the experimental and control groups. You may also conduct multiple posttests at any time during an experiment.

Example:
  1. Are there differences between treatments A and B?
  2. If there is a difference, is it significant or not?
  3. Which treatment is better?

TYPES OF EXPERIMENTAL DESIGNS

Depending on the types of research question and the level of experimental control, a researcher can use different types of experimental designs. The following are descriptions of three major experimental designs:
  1. True Experimental Design
  2. Quasi-Experimental Design
  3. Single-Subject Experimental Design

TRUE EXPERIMENTAL DESIGN

Determines direct influences of the IV on the DV under strictly controlled conditions and permits explicit inferences to be drawn. Subjects are randomly assigned to at least two comparison groups. In true experimental research, the researcher tries to exert maximum control over most of the threats to internal validity, so that she/he can say with confidence that the changes in the DV are a direct result of manipulations of the IV. True experimental designs may be categorized according to how the subjects are assigned to their groups.

1- *Between-Subject Designs or Completely Randomized Designs:* Subjects are assigned to at least two comparison groups using randomization.

2- *Randomized Block Designs:* Subjects are first classified according to a preexisting attribute (block variable) and then on a random basis, the members of each block are assigned to different categories of the independent variable.

Example: The effect of different medications on blood pressure of males and females (block variable). Groups of males and females are each randomly assigned to either experimental (receive medication) or control (no medication) groups, four groups total.

3- *Factorial Designs:* Designs that are described according to the number of independent variables or *factors*, within a design.

    a. Single Factorial Design: Has one independent variable with any number of levels

    b. Two Factorial Design: Has two independent variables with any number of levels

    c. Multi-Factorial Design: Has more than two independent variables with any number of levels

Depending on the number of independent variables and the number of levels for each independent variable (refer to chapter 4), the number of required groups of subjects changes.

For example: A single factorial design has only one IV with at least two levels; therefore, two independent groups of subjects are needed. In two factorial designs, there are two IVs or factors; however, each IV might have different levels. To calculate the number of groups required, the researcher multiplies the levels of each IV.

For example: A 2X2 factorial design means two independent variables with two levels for each IV. This design would require four groups (2X2=4). A 2X3X2 design means 3 independent variables, with the first IV having two levels, the second IV with three levels and the third IV having two levels. This design would need 12 groups of independent subjects that would be randomly assigned to each level of the IVs. As you can see, as the number and levels of IV increases, the design gets more complicated.

Example: What would be the effect of aerobic exercise performed 2 times per week vs. three times per week on blood pressure of a group of patients with high blood pressure? Also, is there a difference in response to exercise if the subjects receive a regular or low fat diet during the exercise?
This is considered a 3X2 factorial design, which will require six randomly assigned groups (3X2=6). There are two independent variables one is exercise (A), with three levels: two times per week, three times per week and no exercise at all (a1, a2, a3). The second independent variable is diet (B), with two levels: low fat diet and regular diet (b1, b2)

Group 1: Exercises 2 times per week, with regular diet
Group 2: Exercises 3 times per week, with regular diet
Group 3: Exercises 2 times per week with diet low in fat
Group 4: Exercises 3 times per week with diet low in fat
Group 5: No exercise with a regular diet (control)
Group 6: No exercise with a low fat diet (control)

The statistical analysis used in factorial designs usually evaluates the ***main effect***, meaning the differences between each IV, independent of the levels, and ***the interaction effects***, meaning the interaction between the different levels of each IV.

The Design Asks the Following Questions:
Are there differential effects between the two IVs?
What is the interaction between the levels of the IVs?

The researcher usually develops a matrix for the statistical analysis.

A

	a1	a2	A3
b1	a1b1	a2b1	a3b1
b2	a1b2	a2b2	a3b2

B

A comparison between A and B evaluates the ***main effect***. What is the overall difference in blood pressure response between those who ate a low fat diet versus a regular diet and exercised 2 times per week and 3 times per week? Comparison between a1b1, a2b1, a1b2, a2 b2, a1a2, b1b2, a3b1, a3b2 evaluates ***the interactions*** (i.e., exercise two times per week with regular diet vs. with diet low in fat, exercise 3 times per week with regular diet vs. diet low in fat, etc).

3-Way Factorial Designs. Examines the main effect of 3 IVs (A, B, and C). It examines the double effects.
A x B
B x C
A x C
Or may examine triple effects.
A x B x C
We may also examine the interaction effects of different levels of each IV.
        a1, a2, b1, b2, c1, c2, and c3

Example:
We can add to the above question, the duration of exercise as a third variable (comparing the effects of 10, 30 or 60 minutes of exercise). The design will be 3X2X3. This design will require 18 independent groups.

QUASI-EXPERIMENTAL DESIGN

Quasi means, having some similarity to, or having some characteristics of. The quasi-experimental design has some resemblance to, and possesses some characteristics of a true experimental design. It is used most of time by clinical researchers who cannot ethically randomly assign subjects into treatment and control groups, or there may not be enough subjects to do randomization. Therefore, the researcher may choose two pre-existing contrasted groups of subjects or use available/convenience samples. The researcher may also use a clinical population available, give a treatment to one and use the other as a control. The design does not involve random selection of subjects or random assignment of subjects to groups due to lack of feasibility in a clinical/field setting. In this situation, the researcher tries to impose whatever control she/he can and be alert of confounding variables.

Some Common Quasi-Experimental Designs

1. *None Equivalent Group Designs:* Rather than using a true control, the researcher tries to find another group that is similar to the experimental group and uses them as a comparison. As you will note, there is no randomization in this process, and the researcher tries to match the characteristics of the experimental group to a similar control group. In this situation the control group is called the "comparison group".

2. *Time Series Analysis:* This is the most popular quasi-experimental design. The researcher examines the changes in the dependant variable over time. A time series can be interrupted (only measure pre and post) or non-interrupted (rate of change over time, using multiple measurements). The researcher tries to capture a number of different events over a longer time period to control for the various threats to validity and reliability. The researcher hopes that by evaluating the data over a longer time period, it will generate stable and reliable findings and tell something about the effects of time itself. As a matter of fact, in this design, the independent variable is usually "time" itself. The researcher usually uses the word "trend" instead of cause.

Example: What would be the functional ability of a group of older adults at 3, 6, and 9 months performing muscle-strengthening exercises? In this question, "time" is an independent variable with repeated measures. Subjects will be followed for nine months and repeated measures will be performed at 3, 6, and 9 months.

3. *Repeated Measures/Within-Subjects Design:* In this design, one group of subjects will be tested under all treatment conditions and each subject acts as his or her own control. This design is also called ***within subject design,*** since subjects are compared to themselves and treatment differences are investigated within a subject across treatment conditions. The advantage of this design is the possibility of controlling for individual differences since all characteristics of the subjects across treatment conditions stay the same. Therefore, differences observed are due to the treatment, not variability across subjects. The major disadvantage of this design is the possibility of ***carry over effects or learning effects***. Subjects may learn from previous treatments and respond differently on the next intervention, or some of the effects from a previous treatment might continue during the next intervention. Therefore, the researcher should be aware of this condition and

make sure that the testing is spaced far enough apart to not allow for carry over or learning effects and close enough to not change the response due to changes in the subjects' characteristics over time.

4. *Crossover Design:* In repeated measures design, subjects are exposed to different conditions. Therefore, there is the potential for the effect of test sequence; that is, the subject's response might be different depending on which test is performed first. Effects such as: fatigue, learning, and carry over could be controlled by using the **Counterbalance** or **Crossover Design.** In counterbalance designs, the order of the testing conditions is randomly assigned to the subjects. Subjects receive each condition in a different order. In crossover designs, the researcher may split the subjects into two groups (if they are tested under two conditions). Half of the subjects receive treatment 1 followed by treatment 2 and the other half receive treatment 2 followed by treatment 1.

SINGLE-SUBJECT EXPERIMENTS

True experimental research requires: a control group, random assignment, and a large number of subjects. This might be impossible in clinical research where each subject is unique and individual responses must be recorded and reported. A true experiment uses average data to generalize to a large population. However, if some subjects respond differently than others, the average data would not reveal these individual responses. Therefore, the clinical researcher does what is called a Single Subject design. It is a repeated collection of information on one or a few subjects (usually less that ten) over time during the application and/or removal of treatments. It documents a particular treatment individualized to the patient with the aim of producing significant changes in a condition. In this design, subjects act as their own control since they are compared before, during, and after the intervention.

Characteristics of Single Subject Design

1- Repeated Measurement. The most important characteristic of a single subject design is the systematic collection of repeated measurements of a behavioral response over time. The intervals are usually frequent and regular (every hour, every day). The behavior response, which is also considered the dependent variable, is called the ***Target Behavior***.

2- Design Phases. The second most important characteristic of a single subject design is the representation of at least two phases: a **baseline phase** (before treatment) usually used as a "control", and an **intervention phase** (during treatment). The **target behavior** is measured during repeated times during both phases. Baseline data provides information regarding "no treatment" or " control", and intervention data provides information regarding changes in target behavior due to the treatment.

Characteristics of the Baseline Phase

There are several characteristics that must be met for the baseline phase of a single subject design, including:

1- Stability (minimum variability). The target behavior's response should be consistent across time. If the target behavior has too much variation, it will be impossible to determine if the changes are due to the intervention or natural fluctuations in the behavior.

2- Trend (stable/unstable). The slope, which shows the rate of change in the behavior, should either continuously go down (decelerating) or up (accelerating) or stay in a steady line without much variation, indicating that the target behavior is not changing. A decelerating target behavior may show deterioration of behavior without any intervention while an accelerating slope may show improvement without any intervention. The entire trend of a target behavior must be identified before the application of the intervention, in order to determine with confidence, that the changes in the target behavior following the intervention is actually due to the intervention and not a trend.

Characteristics of the design phases

There are some characteristics that the must met for both phases of a single subjects design, including:

a) Length of Phases.

One of the most important questions in a single subject design is; how long must the length of each phase be in order to record the changes in the target behavior with confidence? Single subject design provides flexibility for the researcher to decide how long each phase of the design must be, depending on the type of research being performed. As a general rule, the length of both phases as well as the intervals of data collection should be the same during both phases. This will control for potential time related factors such as maturation or learning processes. For example, most of the time a researcher makes a one-week interval for each phase with daily measurements of the target behavior during each phase. The overall purpose is to establish a trend of change over time and possibly identify the maximum response of the target behavior to the intervention. Therefore, the researcher often continues the phase until the target behavior no longer changes. In summary, the length of each phase must be sufficient to capture the changes in the target behavior during both phases of the design.

b) Data Collection.

Data collection in a single subject design is performed in different ways depending upon the types of target behavior being measured. The target behavior might be physiological measures such as blood pressure or heart rate, it may be a functional assessment using a specified tool, it might be muscle strength, range of motion of a joint, time it takes to respond to an intervention, etc. Usually, at least 3-4 data points are required during each phase; however, this might change depending on the target behavior and how often the researcher thinks it is necessary to evaluate the behavior.

c) Techniques for Measuring Target Behavior.
<u>Frequency</u>: Target behavior can be measured depending on the number of occurrences. For example, counting the number of times a patient can do a specific task such as exercise, or the number of time a patient loses control and fell over a period of time.
<u>Duration</u>: Target behaviors can be measured according to how long it lasts. The operational definition of duration is very important. Researchers may define duration differently; however, as long as it is operationally defined it can be measured. For example, a researcher may measure how long a patient stays in one position for one trial and consider that the duration, or she/he may consider the average of three trials and consider that the duration of the target behavior.
<u>Magnitude</u>: Target behavior may be measured using instruments that provide quantitative scores; therefore, researchers can measure the magnitude of change of a target behavior following an intervention. The magnitude of change is important for every situation, whether the researcher is looking for a significant change or a very small change.

For example: A researcher may be evaluating the magnitude of change in a functional scale of a disabled person following an intervention.

DATA ANALYSIS IN SINGLE-SUBJECT DESIGN

Data analysis in a single subject design is based on the evaluation of a target behavior within and between each phase. This allows the researcher to see if the target behavior is changing during each phase and whether significant changes occur following an intervention.

Visual Analysis: This is the type of analysis most often used in a single subject design. Data can be analyzed in terms of *within-phase* and *between-phase* characteristics. *Within-phase* data are described according to stability/variability and trend/direction of change. The comparisons are based on changes in the following characteristics:
1. Level
Change in level refers to a change at the point of intervention. It can be described in terms of the mean or average value of a target behavior within a phase.

2. Trend
Refers to the direction of change within a phase. This can be accelerating, decelerating, or stay stable.

3. Slope of a Trend
Refers to the angle of change at the point of the intervention, or the rate of change.

EXAMPLES OF SINGLE SUBJECT DESIGNS

A= Baseline Phase
B= Intervention Phase

Simple AB

This is the weakest and least scientific of single subject designs. There are only two phases and data are collected during the baseline phase and during the intervention phase (pre-and post-treatment). The researcher cannot say that the changes in the target behavior or during the treatment phase are due to the intervention since there is no control data. There is also no extended post-treatment phase to check maintenance.

ABA Design

This design is also called Reversal/Withdrawal (ABA) design. It is the same as AB but with the addition of a third non-treatment phase. It is usually stronger than AB design. Ethical issues may arise with this design; for example, it may be unethical to withdraw treatment if it is medically necessary or if the target behavior response is to the advantage of the patient (do you want to discontinue something that is working?). However, since no baseline data are collected, it can make it hard to evaluate the positive effects.

- *A-B Design*

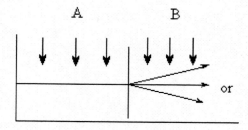

- *ABA Design*

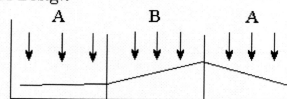

BAB Design

In this design, treatment is instituted, withdrawn, and then re-instituted again. This design can be very effective when therapy must start immediately. The researcher starts the treatment and evaluates the target behavior over time and then withdraws the treatment. If the subject's response is not positive, the treatment is reinstated and the researcher may conclude that the treatment was effective.

There are many more ways that the single subject design could be performed, such as ABAB, BABA, ABACAB (addition of a third treatment C).

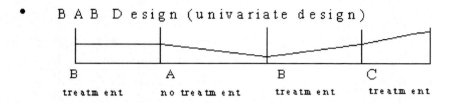

- BAB Design (univariate design)

| B | A | B | C |
| treatment | no treatment | treatment | treatment |

EXPERIMENTAL DESIGNS TO AVOID

One-Group Posttest
Treatment ---> Measurement 1
This is when a researcher chooses a group, gives them the intervention, and measures the dependent variable. This is one of the weakest experimental designs as there is no control group involved. Researchers could hardly prove that any changes that occurred are due to the intervention, or due to chance.

Posttest Designs with Nonequivalent Groups
Experimental group:
  Treatment ---> Measurement 1
Control group
  No treatment --->Measurement 1
In this design, since there is no random assignment of the subjects to groups, subjects may be different in some important ways and their response to the intervention may not be due to the intervention, but due to individual variability.

One-Group Pretest-Posttest
Measurement 1--->Treatment--->Measurement 2
No control group
In this design, again since no control group is involved, we could not attribute the changes to the independent variable. For example, the changes may be due to maturation, development, and history of the subjects.

NOTES

CHAPTER

10

OTHER DESIGN STRATEGIES

OVERALL OBJECTIVE

Develop an understanding of evaluation and epidemiological research and how they are used.

GOALS

1. Develop an understanding of evaluation research
2. Differentiate between different types of evaluation processes
3. Develop an understanding of epidemiological research
4. Differentiate between different epidemiological definitions and concepts
5. Recognize different design strategies for epidemiological research

EVALUATION RESEARCH

In educational or clinical settings, sometimes evaluation tools are developed and implemented to improve the effectiveness, efficiency, and impact of a new program or policy. Program evaluation is defined as the use of a research approach to measure the effects of a program in terms of its goals, outcomes, or criteria. The results of evaluation research may be used to improve or develop new policy-oriented programming. This type of research, although it is introducing new interventions and appears to be like experimental research, has major differences with experimental design.

For example: Assume that you are the director of a health promotion program in a large company. The company asks you to develop a nutrition intervention program to improve the heath of the employees. You may propose an educational program that will teach the employees about making good food choices, how to increase their consumption of fruits and vegetables and reduce their consumption of fatty and junk foods. You will have some outcome measures or indicators that your program is making progress and that the employees are making changes in their behavior. Your program will involve: you as the program coordinator, a nutritionist, and maybe the supervisors of the dinning facility to work with you and provide the proper choices for the employees. This example is considered evaluation research. The results of such a program may be used to change the company's policy on food preparation or on providing health care.

Differences Between Evaluation Research and Experimental Research

1- Program evaluation is a clear example of applied research, meaning that you are looking at the immediate effect of a program in your setting. You would also use the results as a base for future decision making as to whether to continue the program or not. Experimental research mostly tries to explain the underlying phenomenon or theory without looking at its immediate effect.

2- Program evaluation usually is performed following a needs assessment. The company or institution will first develop some plan to evaluate whether or not such a program is necessary. Following the needs assessment, they will develop a program to deal with problems that may surface during the needs assessment. In the example above, the company might have realized that the health insurance of the employees is high and after the needs assessment found that the majority of the employees are over the age 50 years and are overweight. Based on this information, they propose a nutrition intervention program. In clinical research you do not need to do a need assessments.

3- The program, which is like an intervention in experimental research, is subject to change during the course of the evaluation. In experimental research, you have to plan everything in advance, once you start the intervention no change is allowed. In program evaluation, the researcher performs what is called a **Process Evaluation.** During the process evaluation, if it was found that something has to be changed to increase the program's effectiveness, it will be incorporated, even if you are in the middle of the program. For instance, in the example above, if in the midst of the program evaluation, it is found that dining services involvement is not as high as desired, adjustments may be made to increase their involvement. There is also another component called **Impact Evaluation**. This component evaluates the progress toward the ultimate goal of the project/program. What impact has the program had so far in the population under investigation? In our example, periodic weight or body mass index may be collected to see if employees have lost weight. The combination of process evaluation and impact evaluation is called **Formative Evaluation.** At the completion of the program, the coordinator may collect some data to evaluate how well the program attained its major goals. This evaluation is called **Summative Evaluation** and is usually the final report of the project that contains information about the long-term benefits of the program and the population it impacts. In our example, the employees of a large company.

Overall, evaluation research is a complex and specialized form of applied research. During the process of evaluation, the researcher may use descriptive, correlation or other types of statistical analysis such as t-tests or analysis of variance. The most important issues are to identify the variables of interest, to realize what indicators must be measured and at what point in time to evaluate the program.

EPIDEMIOLOGICAL RESEARCH

The fundamental goal of epidemiological research studies is to improve the overall health of the public. It is the study of health and disease that includes: determining the frequency of disease and health status, determining factors that effect the development or progress of specific health problems and their trends, predicting the probability of occurrence of specific diseases or conditions, and finally, determining factors that prevent diseases, improves health, and prolongs life. The majority of information that we have today regarding epidemiology of infectious disease, the importance of clean water supplies, and food refrigeration are the direct result of epidemiological studies. Relationships that have been established between disease and environmental conditions such as smoking and lung cancer, or sun exposure and melanoma are also part of epidemiological studies.

Terms in Epidemiological Studies

1. Exposure: This also called *causal factors.* They reflect life style practices such as smoking, occupational hazards such as repetitive motions, or environmental influences such as sun exposure that may cause a disease or health condition.

2. Risk Factors: Risk factors are conditions that, if exposed to, may increase or decrease the likelihood of developing or not developing certain disorders or conditions. For example, smoking is a risk factor for developing lung cancer.

3. Prevalence (P): This is reflected as the proportion of existing cases of a disorder relative to the total population at a given point in time. It is an estimate of the probability that an individual may have a certain disease and is calculated as:

$$P = \frac{\text{Number of existing cases of a disease at a given point in time}}{\text{Total population at risk}}$$

4. Incidence Rate (IR): The estimate of the risk of developing new cases of a disorder or disease in the population during a specified time period. It can be calculated as:

$IR=$ <u>Number of new cases during a given time period</u>
Total person-time

Person-time is the sum of the time periods of observation for all individuals in the population at risk during the study's time frame.

5. *Cumulative Incidence (CI)*: The number of individuals who become diseased during a specified time period and is calculated as:

$CI=$ <u>Number of new cases during a given time period</u>
Total population at risk

The difference between the IR and CI is that in the IR the denominator is the total number of people observed during a specific time, while the denominator in the CI is measuring and following the entire population at risk during a specific time period. This is harder and more time consuming than IR.

6. *Birth Rate and Mortality Rate:* Epidemiologists may measure the health status of a population in terms of birth and death rates and morbidity. They are calculated as follows:

Birth Rate= <u>Number of live births in one year</u>
Total population in midyear

Mortality Rate= <u>Number of deaths in one year</u>
Total population at midyear

Case specific death = <u>Number of deaths from a particular disease in one year</u>
Average midyear population

Case fatality rate= <u>Number of deaths from a particular disease in one year</u>
Number of people who had the disease in that year

Morbidity rate= <u>Number of people who get the disease in one year</u>
Total population in midyear

7. *Attributable Risk (AR):* The absolute effect of a specific exposure could be determined by looking at the differences in frequency of the disease for those who were exposed and unexposed. The difference between the incidence of disease in the exposed and unexposed is called *Attributable risk.*

8. *Relative Risk (RR):* It is the likelihood that someone that has been exposed to a risk factor will develop the disease as compared to somebody who has not been exposed.

Epidemiologists use the above calculations to estimate and predict a population's health status at any time. The major distinction of epidemiological studies is that a large sample of the population is usually studied and inferences are made based on the collected data to the population as a whole. An epidemiologist may use descriptive/observational, correlational, or experimental approaches to answer their questions. In ***observational or descriptive epidemiological studies***, the epidemiologist observes the population without any manipulation in order to study the distribution, pattern, or trend of a disease or disability in a population.

Descriptive epidemiological studies are done in situations where little is known about the occurrence or determinants of a specific health condition. In ***correlational epidemiological studies,*** the epidemiologist tries to establish relationships between a disease and a particular risk factor or exposure. Usually the epidemiologist routinely uses data available from large databases developed by government or private health organizations and tries to establish the relationships or trends. The major limitation of correlational studies is that it cannot establish a cause and effect relationship.

In *Case-Control studies*, an epidemiologist may choose a group who has a disease and compare them to a group without the disease. The epidemiologist then may go backwards and study both groups as far as their exposures, using questionnaires, interviews, or reviewing charts to collect as much data as possible on both groups. Their assumption is that differences in past exposures or lifestyles might have caused one group to acquire the disease and the other not too. This a retrospective approach to establish a cause and effect relationship.

The most common experimental approach in epidemiological research is *randomized clinical trials*. This a prospective approach to establish a cause and effect relationship by comparing an experimental group who receives an intervention with a control group who will not. The subjects are randomly assigned to either an experimental or control group. This design has the strongest internal and external validity due to random selection and assignment of the subjects. The number of subjects is usually large. For example, a clinician might be comparing two different treatment approaches for his or her cancer patients. She/he may randomly assign subjects to receive one or the other treatment for 5 years and follow up with them after the treatments to see which group is doing better.

Non-randomized clinical trials are usually performed on studies of community intervention programs. Some type of intervention may be provided for a community and the results are compared with another community that did not receive the intervention. For example, a new diabetes education program may be offered to an African American community to teach awareness of the early signs of the disease and how to control the disease after onset. After 5 years, the prevalence and incidence of the disease in this community can be compared with another community that did not receive the intervention. If the incidence and prevalence rate is significantly less in the intervention group, the researcher may conclude that the intervention was effective and should be offered to other similar communities.

SUMMARY

Program evaluation and epidemiological research provide different approaches to answer clinical research questions. Although it seems overwhelming to consider all the research approaches available to a researcher, choosing one approach over the other is the most important part of the research planning process. The choice should be based on the nature of the research question, the availability of subjects and resources, and the knowledge of the researcher.

EXERCISES FOR CHAPTERS 9-10

1- *Instructions:* For each of the following research studies, indicate whether the experimental procedures that were carried out were correct or incorrect, ethical or unethical. Explain why?
   a. A clinician was looking for subjects and 60 of his patients volunteered to participate in an experiment. The clinician then randomly assigned 30 of them to an experimental group and 30 of them to a control group.
   b. A teacher is planning an experiment to test the effectiveness of a new teaching program to 10th grade math students. In order to prevent bias from entering into the experiment, the teacher decides not to give a pretest prior to starting the experiment.

2- Design an experiment using ABA design.

3-When subjects are divided at random, what type of experiment is being conducted?

4-What is the major purpose of an experiment?

5-What does quasi-experimental research mean and what are the different types?

6- Suppose, as part of a program evaluation, an evaluator asks at the conclusion of a health promotion program, "How many employees are participating in the fitness club activities?" Is this question relevant to formative, summative, or impact evaluation?

QUESTIONS FOR DISCUSSION

1- Have you ever carried out an experiment by introducing a treatment to a person or a group and measured the effect(s) on the dependent variable(s)? If so, briefly describe. Do you think you would you have had better information if you had included a control group? Explain.

2- A program director wants to evaluate her program in the best possible way. Would an internal reviewer be better than an external one? Why?

3- Suppose you want to know if playing classical music during the class has a positive effect on students' behavior and attention. Would you do an experimental research study or a non-experimental? Why?

4- Assume that a physician is treating a patient with a severe type of cancer. The side effects of the cancer treatment is causing the patient to lose her appetite and get weaker everyday. The doctor is not sure whether the cancer treatment is working or if he should continue with the treatment. What type of research can this doctor do to answer the questions? Why?

FOR STUDENTS WHO ARE PLANNING TO DO RESEARCH

Have you identified your research design? If yes, what type of design is most appropriate to answer your research question and why?

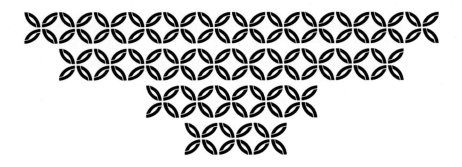

NOTES

PART IV

MEASUREMENTS IN RESEARCH

CHAPTER (11)   Principals of Measurement
CHAPTER (12)   Reliability of Measurements
CHAPTER (13)   Validity of Measurements

CHAPTER

11

PRINCIPALS OF MEASUREMENT

OVERALL OBJECTIVE

Become familiar with the terms and concepts associated with measuring and defining study data.

GOALS

1- Illustrate the principles of measurement
2- Understand the rules of measurements
3- Recognize different levels of measurements and their applications

PRINCIPLES OF MEASUREMENT

Measurement is the assignment of numerals to objects, representing quantities of characteristic(s,) or attribute(s) for better understanding, evaluating, differentiating, and communicating the characteristics of people, objects, events, that are the focus of an investigation. Measurement helps to communicate information in objective terms, giving a sense of "how much" or "how little". It also allows for levels of precision when describing characteristics according to their quantity, degree, quality, etc. For example, instead of saying, "today is hotter than yesterday," you say "the temperature is 98° Fahrenheit today vs. 87° yesterday". As you can see with the first sentence, the audience has no idea about how hot the temperature is, whereas in the second sentence, you have a better **understanding** of how hot it is!

In another example, you may say "the patient is feeling better today", rather than saying "I evaluated the range of motion in the patient's joint and it has increased 10 degrees compared to yesterday. He has no pain and, therefore, is feeling better". The latter sentences made you **evaluate** how the patient feels better, while the first sentence does not give you any indication or basis for the evaluation.

In another example, you may say, "those who perform better on their exam will be allowed to go to the next level" or you may say "students are required to get a passing grade of B or above in order to move to the next level". The second sentence allow you to **discriminate** between two conditions. There are three basic processes in measurement: *conceptualization, operationalization and determination.*

Conceptual Definition: Many times a researcher is measuring a construct or concept. The researcher must define this construct and find a conceptual or theoretical definition that explains it. These conceptual definitions are completely different than dictionary definitions and must be definitions that others in the scientific community agree on. The majority of the time, the researcher finds the same conceptualization used by others from the literature and uses that. Sometimes, if the concept is something absolutely new, researchers may come up with their own definitions. However, one must make sure that the definition is understandable and agreeable by the scientific community.

Operational Definition: One of the most important steps in measurement is to operationally define the variables that you are trying to measure and determine how you will be measuring them. During this process, the researcher defines the concept and makes it more precise to the point that it can be measured. This process is called finding operational definitions, or finding concrete indicators of measuring the concept. Unless you know what the term means, you cannot show that it exists. Variables can be measured either directly (i.e., height, weight) or indirectly (i.e., temperature, measuring the length of the change in a mercury tube). Some variables are constructs such as intelligence or stress. Measurement of a construct is based on the expectation of how a person who possesses the specific trait would behave in certain situations. For example, if you operationally define "psychological health" during your operationalization, you should not be measuring social health or physical health. Your definition and measurements must be able to discriminate between these concepts. The most important issue is your unit of analysis. You must make sure that throughout the research process all the measurements are reduced to the same unit of analysis for the specific variable. For example, if you are measuring subjects' weight, you must make sure that if you use pounds as your unit of analysis, the entire groups' weight must be taken in pounds, not in kilograms or anything else.

Determination: This is the process of determining the levels of measurement, and then even more advanced methods of measuring the reliability and validity of measurements.

MEASUREMENTS APPLICATIONS

Measurement is the assignment of numerals to objects. A numeral is a symbol, which has no quantitative meaning (i.e., 1=Male, 2=Female or 1=Yes, 2=No).

Measurement may be used as a continuous variable, which can take on any value along a continuum (i.e., 1 - 10), or it may used as discrete variable, which describes things only in whole units (heart rate, number of steps taken during walking).

Precision is the number of decimals used in the measurement. The higher the number of decimals, the higher the precision of the measurement system will be. For example, the researcher may measure a person's height only as a whole number or he may use up to one or two decimals.

Overall Use of Measurements in Research
1. To describe the quality or quantity of an existing variable
2. To make a decision based on a criterion or standard of performance
3. As a basis for choosing between two courses of action
4. To evaluate conditions and responses to treatment
5. To compare individuals or groups
6. To draw conclusions about predictive relationships between variables

RULES OF MEASUREMENT

The rules of measurements are the establishment of purposeful and precise rules for assigning values to objects. The researcher must stay within those rules throughout the duration of the research. After you define your variable, identify the measurement system and units to be used, you have to follow those rules otherwise the data collected is meaningless.

The rules should:
1. Designate how numbers are to be assigned
2. Reflect the amount and the unit of measurement
3. Define the variable and explain the difference between values
4. Provide the basis for a measurement system to appreciate how the rules can be applied
5. Ensure that the rules apply to the acceptable operations with which numerals can be manipulated

LEVELS OF MEASUREMENT

Rules of measurement are also applied to how a numeral could be manipulated and what types of mathematical operations could be used to evaluate it. For example, not all the variables could be divided or multiplied, some may only be used as a frequency count. The nature of the attribute being measured dictates the rule(s) that can be used to measure it. There are four levels of measurement scales that, depending on the types of variables under investigation, could be used by a researcher: *nominal, ordinal, interval, and ratio.* The ratio measurement is the highest level of measurement, offering more flexibility for mathematical operations.

Nominal Scale: In this scale, numbers represent categories only, and are used purely as labels for identification. You should not do any arithmetical operations with nominal data; only count the number in each category. This is considered the weakest level of measurement and least precise. When categories are assigned, they must be discrete and exclusive, independent (all different and unrelated), and exhaustive (must fit into one category).

Examples: -Yes   - No
              - Male - Female

The researcher counts the number of males or females in the study or counts the number of times the subjects answer yes or no.

Ordinal Scale: In this category, data are assigned symbols in order to rank them. The intervals between the ranks may not be known as the data represents a position within a distribution. The position within the distribution is always the same; however, the difference between the two positions is not the same. For example, a researcher may categorize muscle tone from 0 (no tone) to 4 (maximum tone). If Subject (1) is graded 2 and Subject (2) is graded 4 on this scale, this does not means that Subject 2 has twice the muscle tone as Subject 1.

The categories assigned may have a true zero, or an arbitrary zero. Sometimes the researcher may evaluate subjects based on having or not having an attribute and assign a number as the middle ground. The responses could move away in both directions. For example, a researcher may ask the subjects' opinion about an issue and give the subjects the choice of: disagree, neutral, and agree. This type of scale cannot be manipulated with arithmetical operations and is only appropriate for descriptive analysis (i.e., frequency count).

Examples:

Tone: (none--minimal--moderate--severe)

Level of physical activity: (good--fair--poor)

Attitude: (strongly agree--agree--disagree)

Metric Scale: In metric scales, the distance between any two numbers on the scale is known and equal in size. Real numbers are assigned to quantifiably evaluate the subjects. This type of scale allows arithmetical operations. There are two categories within this scale:

1. *Interval:* This scale does not have a true zero point. Either the researcher defines an arbitrary zero for this scale and any number within the system will be evaluated against that zero, or there already exists scales that researcher can use. In both situations, data can be added and subtracted, but these operations cannot be used to interpret actual quantities because the results cannot be logically measured against true zero. For example, the years 1999 and 2000 are interval level of measurement because we are measuring the passage of time against an arbitrary zero (B.C., or A.D). When we say the year is 2002, this does not mean that the beginning of the life was 2002 years ago. Temperature is another example of an interval level of measurement. For the centigrade system, 0° is the temperature at which water freezes, while the

freezing point on the Fahrenheit scale is 32°. However, in both scales, the difference between the two temperatures is the same, meaning that if you change the temperature from 70° to 80° the difference is always 10 degrees.

2. *Ratio:* In this type of measurement scale, there is an absolute zero. This is the highest level of measurement and values can be manipulated by addition, subtraction, multiplication, and division. For example, height, weight, and force are ratio measurements, since you are measuring their values against true zero.

Remember that as a researcher you must define the rules of measurement and based on your research question set the rules for measuring a variable.

Example: We measured the length of 4 tables and presented the data using the 4 levels of measurement. Typically, the highest level of measurement in this situation would be the ratio scale since we have a true zero; however; we can illustrate how you can use other scales.

Table	Nominal	Ordinal	Interval	Ratio
1	Long	2	30	240
2	Long	3	60	270
3	Short	1	0	210
4	Long	4	100	310

The first column describes the data using a nominal scale. We said any table 210 cm or lower is (SHORT) and greater than 210 cm is LONG (*operational definition*). Therefore, we will have only two categories (SHORT and LONG) consisting of one SHORT and three LONGS. Since categories are assigned by numerals, we do not know the difference between the three longs. In the second column, we used an ordinal scale and made the rule that the lowest number in the distribution is (1) and the next higher number is (2) and so on----. In this scale, we end up with four numbers, which identifies the position of each table's length within the distribution. In this scale, even though we know table number four has the longest length, we do not know exactly by how much. In the third column, we used an interval scale, setting the shortest table length of 210 cm as zero and measuring the rest of the table lengths according to this arbitrary zero. In this category, we know the difference between each table's lengths; however, we do not know the exact length of each table. The last column shows a ratio measurement scale, which is the best way to measure the table length with a true zero.

Measurement Operations. Nominal and ordinal data can only be described by frequency counts. Interval data can be added or subtracted. Ratio data can be added, subtracted, multiplied, and divided. Tests of statistical inferences that require arithmetical manipulation can only be applied to interval or ratio data.

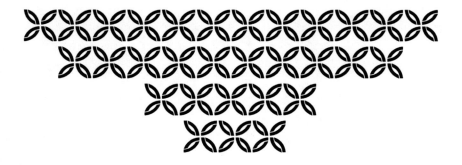

NOTES

CHAPTER

12

RELIABILITY

OVERALL OBJECTIVE

Develop an understanding of measurement characteristics and the importance of reliability of the measurements during the conduct of research.

GOALS

1. Identify different sources of error in the measurements and measurement systems
2. Learn how to control the error in the measurements
3. Develop an understanding of the concept of reliability and how to test it

MEASUREMENT CHARACTERISTICS

For a study to be accurate, its finding must be **reliable** (dependable), **objective** (confirmable) and **valid** (credible). These are the three main prerequisites for interpreting the results of any research study and will be discussed in this chapter.

Reliability is the degree of consistency in which a test measures what it is supposed to measure. It is the ability of a test to measure the same thing repeatedly and get the same results consistently (reproducibility). It is the extent to which a measurement is consistent and free from error. Therefore, reliability is the same as dependability and predictability. In order to understand reliability, one needs to understand errors in measurement.

Measurement Error. There is always some error in measurement such that the true scores take into account some level of error;

X (Observed score) = T (True score) + E (Error measurement)

Reliability is estimating how much of our measurement is due to error and how much is an accurate reading.

Types of Measurement Error

Measurement errors can be *systematic or random*. *Systematic errors*, or predictable errors of measurement, are errors that can be corrected by the researcher. It is when a measurement system consistently over estimates or under estimates the true score. For example, imagine a measuring tape that is 2 inches short. For every data point measured with this tape, the researcher must add 2 inches to correct this systematic error.

Random errors are due to chance and are unpredictable errors of measurement. They are called chance errors as they can unpredictably affect a subject's score. These errors could be due to the tester, the measurement system, or a subject may contribute to them. For example, if you are asked to measure the heights of a group of thirty people. One of the sources of error might be you as the tester. As you continue with your testing; even though for the first few subjects you paid significant attention to the procedures of your testing (i.e., proper positioning of the subjects, and the measuring tape, shoes off, etc.), after a while you may not follow the procedures properly, either due to fatigue, boredom, or many other factors and report subjects data incorrectly. Another source of error might be the instrument that is used for testing. In this case, the measuring tape. It is possible that after so many uses the tape stretches out, or if you are doing your testing on different days, there might be environmental conditions that affect the measuring tape's performance (over stretched or under stretched). As a result, you may get incorrect readings and again report inaccurate data. The last source of error that may affect the measurements is the subjects themselves. They may get fatigued, become uncooperative, and may not follow the procedures. This is the hardest source of error to control, since you never know if the subjects are performing at their optimal level. As you can see there are many sources of error in the measurements and, as a researcher, you must be aware of these sources and try to control them as much as possible.

One way to control for measurement error is through reliability testing.

ESTIMATE OF RELIABILITY

Reliability is the extent to which test scores are free from error or the extent to which the scores vary from the true scores. The estimation of reliability is based on the statistical concept of *variance*. Because we never know the exact true measure, we estimate reliability through the variability of the scores within the same sample. The less variable the scores are, the more reliable the test will be. For example, if you want to see if a measuring tape is a reliable instrument for measuring height, you may measure the height of ten people at two different times. In those measurements, there will be some variance (differences) in the heights of the subjects, which is a true difference. There are also some variances that are due to sources of error that were explained above (tester, measuring tape, or subject). The more homogenous the data is, the less variability exists in the true scores, and the less error variance, the more reliable the measuring tape would be. Therefore, reliability is a measure of how much of the total variance is attributed to the true difference between scores and how much is attributed to error. This is expressed as the Reliability Coefficient.

RC = Reliability Coefficient: Is a mathematical estimation of reliability. It is the ratio between the true score variance and the true score variance plus error variance.

$$\frac{true\ score\ variance}{true\ score\ variance + error\ variance}$$

Magnitude of RC:

RC = 1   (Perfect Reliability)
    RC = 0 (No Reliability)

An RC of 1 means perfect reliability, which is hardly ever true as it means there is no error variance. An RC of 0 means that the test is not reliable at all, which is also rare. Therefore, most researchers assume some level of acceptability for the RC. For example, an RC of 0.50 or lower may be considered "not acceptable", an RC of 0.50-0.75 may be considered "moderate reliability", and the values above 0.75 may be considered "good reliability".

Correlation and Agreement

The tests for reliability measures are based on the measurement of the *correlation coefficient*. Correlation is the degree of association between two sets of data, or consistency in the position of each data point within the distribution. For example, if you measure the height and step length of a group of ten people, you may find that there is a high correlation between height and step length. In other words, those who are taller take longer steps. Reliability could be interpreted in the same way. A measuring tape is a reliable instrument if you measure a group of ten people twice and the tallest person in the first set is also the tallest in the second set. In this test you find a high correlation between the two sets of data and assume the tape is a reliable measurement system. However, there is another component that needs to be considered when using correlation for reliability testing and that is the agreement between the data points. We have to prove that not only the highest scores in the first data set are the highest in the second, but also that they are the same or not significantly different (random source of errors). This is called **agreement** and the statistical analysis used to determine agreement is called *interclass correlation coefficient (ICC)*. ICC not only looks at the consistency in the positioning of the scores within the distribution, but also evaluates the level of agreement between two sets of scores.

TYPES OF RELIABILITY

Source of Measurement Error. As it was discussed before, there are basically three sources of error within each measurement system: the person performing the test (rater), the instrument utilized to measure the variable (instrument), and the subjects who are under investigation. To test the reliability of a test, one must assume the other two components are reliable/consistent. For example, to test the reliability of a tester you must have a reliable instrument and subjects. Or, to test the reliability of an instrument, you must make sure that your rater and subjects are reliable. Depending on the type of research being conducted, sometimes the researcher may have to record the reliability of one of these components.

RATER RELIABILITY

The validity of any study depends on the reliability of the tester. Data cannot be interpreted with confidence unless those who collect, record and reduce it are reliable. There are different ways that one could establish the reliability of a rater.

I. Intra-Rater Reliability. This is establishing the reliability of data recorded across two or more trials by one rater. This is for situations where only one rater is collecting all of the data. It is usually established by having one tester perform multiple trials (more than one) on the same group of subjects and then examining to see if he or she is consistently getting the same results. Many researchers establish intra-rater reliability by having one experienced rater do all the rating and then assume the rater is reliable due to personal experience.

II. Inter-Rater Reliability. Inter-rater reliability is establishing the reliability of data collected between two or more raters who measure the same group of subjects. Sometimes, due to the research protocol, more that one person is responsible for subject testing. Inter-rater reliability establishes the consistency of measurements taken by two or more raters. Usually, the raters test the subjects at the same time. This is very hard to do in situations where there is a possibility of carry over, learning effect, or fatigue in the subjects. It can be done in situations where both raters simultaneously observe the subjects and rate them for some characteristic at the same time. For example, having two different raters look through a mirrored glass and rate the subjects' performance individually and then evaluate their reported data to see of they both collected consistent data on these subjects. Because establishing inter-rater reliability is hard, researchers usually control for this by using only one rater for all of the testing.

INSTRUMENT RELIABILITY

Reliability of an instrument could be established in three ways:
I.   Test/Retest Reliability

II.   Equivalence
III.   Internal Consistency

I. Test/Retest Reliability.
This test establishes that an instrument is capable of measuring a variable with consistency over time. One sample group is tested under the same conditions, using an identical test, two or more different times. Keeping all testing conditions equal, if the test is reliable, the subjects' score should be similar after multiple trials. The coefficient derived from this testing is called the *test-retest reliability coefficient.*

When responses are changing (i.e., increase in muscle strength over time, healing process), test-retest reliability may be impossible to determine. Sometimes the rater is part of the measurement system and the test- retest reliability is performed to see if the tester is producing the same results under the same conditions. For example, a physical therapist who is measuring the patients' muscle tone. He or she is the actual measurement system. This is a subjective rating of the patients muscle tone (0 (no tone) - 4 (maximum tone). You have to establish his/her reliability of recording muscle tone.

Test-Retest Reliability is affected by...
A. Testing Effect: The first test may affect the outcome of the second test either due to learning; carry over, fatigue, etc.
Example: In testing a subject's muscle tone, repeated testing may cause the subject's tone to get better or worse.

B. Test-Retest Intervals: In test-retest reliability, the stability of the response under investigation is very important. Therefore, time intervals between each test must be considered very carefully. Usually, the tests should be far enough apart to avoid fatigue or learning and close enough to avoid changes in the measured variable.

C. Rater Bias: When one rater is involved in both test and retest, the memory of the first score can influence the recording of the second score. The rater may remember a subject's score from the first measurement and just record it on the next trial. This error can be corrected by either blinding the tester to the results of the first test, or by developing objective grading criteria and training the tester. Rater bias is very hard to control in situations where the tester is an integral part of the measurement system.

II. Equivalence = Alternate Forms of Reliability.
This is performed in situations where, the researcher is interested in establishing the reliability of two measurement instruments, which measures the same response (parallel reliability). For example, we all know that the SAT is offered four or five times per year. All of these tests are supposed to test the students' knowledge in different subjects. How do we know that each SAT is measuring the same thing? To establish the reliability of these tests, the researcher performs *equivalence or alternate* forms of reliability testing. To do the reliability testing, usually two alternative forms of these tests are given to the same group of students in one

sitting. Those who receive high grades in one test must also receive high grades on the other one. By establishing the equivalence, absolute values are compared or equated across tests to generalize findings from one study to another or from research to practice.

III.   Internal Consistency/Homogeneity.   This type of reliability is established for instruments such as questionnaires and written exams that are designed to measure particular knowledge. It reflects the extent to which items measure the same characteristics. If test items are reliable, they should reflect the test taker's true score. There are two ways to establish this type of reliability:

A- Split-Half Reliability: Is a measuring technique that is used to check the internal consistency of an educational testing instrument (i.e., exams). One group of subjects take a test composed of twice as many items as needed, with half the items being redundant of the other half.
Items are then divided into two comparable halves for scoring. If each subject's half-test scores are correlated, the whole test is considered reliable. This controls for the physical, mental, and environmental influences that will affect the subjects during testing.

B- Test Item Reliability: Assesses internal consistency by conducting an item analysis. It examines how each item on a test relates to every other item or to the instrument as a whole. Those who respond well on one item would respond well on the test as a whole.
For example, if a professor wants to give a reliable exam to his/her students, he/she may use test item reliability by identifying different components of the course and scoring students on each component. The students will also have a total score for the whole exam. Students who score the highest on the whole exam would have also scored the highest on each of the items making up the exam.

SUBJECT RELIABILITY

Subjects under study also play a role on the reliability of the tests. If subjects are not reliable, even with a reliable tester and instrument, the data will be meaningless. Sometimes the subject's characteristics are changeable, due to either environmental conditions or human response, such as motivation, fatigue, and cooperation. Sometimes the response under study is fluctuating. For example, blood pressure in one subject fluctuates from time to time even without any intervention. These types of subject fluctuations are hard to control and their contribution to error may not be controllable.

NOTES

CHAPTER

13

VALIDITY

OVERALL OBJECTIVE

Develop an understanding of the importance of test validity in research.

GOALS

1. Understand the difference between validity and reliability
2. Identify different types of test validity and their applications

VALIDITY

Validity is the degree to which an instrument measures what it is assumed to measure. It is the appropriateness, truthfulness, authenticity, and effectiveness of a study. It is the extent to which measurement is useful for making decisions relevant to a given response.

Validity, to a large extent, depends on the logic and rational of the research design. To establish the validity of a test, one must be able to answer the following questions:

1. Is the test capable of *discriminating* among individuals with and without specific characteristics?
2. Can the test *evaluate* the magnitude of change over time?
3. Can the test be used to *predict* a potential outcome?
If the answer is yes, then the test is a valid test.

Validity and Reliability

The fact that an instrument is measuring something consistently *does not* mean that it is measuring what we want it to measure.

Reliability is a prerequisite to validity, but a reliable test may not be a valid test. For example, if somebody uses a measuring tape to evaluate back pain, no matter how reliable the measuring tape is, it is not a valid test for measuring back pain. On the other hand, if an unreliable measuring tape is used to measure the step length of a group of subjects as part of the data collection, the data collected is not valid. For a test to be valid it has to be reliable. Depending on the type of research and the types of tests being used, a researcher may or may not have to establish the validity of a test. Some instruments are obvious for measuring a specific response and a researcher does not have to establish its validity. However, sometimes a researcher must come up with his/her own instrument to measure a response. In this situation she/he must first establish the validity of the test/instrument.

TEST VALIDITY

1. "Face Validity". This is the lowest level of validity testing. By establishing the face validity of an instrument, the researcher is basically saying that this instrument appears to measure what it is supposed to measure and this is a credible method for doing it. This is considered the weakest form of validity, and is used for situations where the instrument is the only one of its kind and no other instrument can be found for comparison. It is mainly based on the judgment of the investigator. Some instruments have face validity inherent in them and are accepted in the scientific community as a valid measurement system for a specific test. Under these circumstances, the researcher does not have to establish their validity. For example, we all know that a goniometer measures angles in degrees and joints are like angles, a goniometer could be used to measure the range of motion of a joint. As the range of motion increases, the goniometer's angle increases.

One of the most important factors in face validity is that those who use the test and those who are being tested must agree that this is a valid test. For example, if the scientific community does not agree with an instrument that an investigator has used to measure a variable, the data collected is useless. The subjects' acceptance of a test is also important, as the test must relate to something that the subjects understand to ensure better cooperation. It should be noted that even though face validity is the weakest type of validity, it is a prerequisite for all other types of validity.

2. "Content Validity". Content validity indicates that the items that make up an instrument, adequately sample the universe of content that defines the variable being measured. The investigator asks, "Does this test truly sample the behavior that I want to study?" Content validity is an important part of questionnaires, examinations, and interviews that attempt to evaluate a range of information by selected test items. For example, assume that a professor who is teaching a Research Methodology course, wants to give an exam to measure the students' "*knowledge of Research Methodology*" based on the course lectures. There are many questions that she/he can choose from to test the students' *knowledge*; however, she/he chooses 40 questions out of all the possible questions. We can say that this exam has content validity and is a valid instrument to measure the "*knowledge in Research Methodology*" if it accurately measures all the universe of content that defines the variable ("*knowledge in Research Methodology*"). Another important component of content validity is that a test should only measure the variable of interest and nothing else. A test of "*knowledge in Research Methodology*" should not measure the *knowledge of Mathematical Concepts.*

In order to establish the content validity, the investigator first chooses the instrument and then may ask a panel of "experts" in the area to examine the instrument and see if this is a valid test for measuring the variable under investigation. In other words, content validity is like face validity, with the difference being that content validity is a post hoc form of validation and judgment is made after an instrument is constructed.

3- "Criterion Related Validity". This is one of the most useful methods to establish the validity of an instrument. It is based on predictive ability of one test for the results on another test. The researcher usually chooses an instrument, which is cheaper, safer, or more practical (***the target test***) and establishes its validity by comparing it with an already established instrument (***gold standard or criterion***).

For example, we know that the ***gold standard*** instrument for measuring leg length is X-ray evaluation of the lower limb. However, this is a costly instrument and may expose the subjects to unnecessary radiation. The researcher then chooses a measuring tape as a ***target*** test and establishes its validity by comparing the results with the X-ray, which is the gold standard. To establish this validity, the researcher may choose a group of subjects and measure them once with the X-Ray and then once with the measuring tape. By achieving comparable results, she/he establishes the validity of the measuring tape as an instrument for measuring leg length.

There are some specific characteristics that must be met by the criterion measure:

1- The most important criteria for the criterion or gold standard is that it has to be reliable and valid. If these two components are not met, it is a useless gold standard.
2- The gold standard and the target test must be independent from each other and free from bias. For example, using a supervisor's rating of the workers as the "*gold standard*" for validating a scale that measures workers performance. There is a possibility of bias in this gold standard.
3- The last and most important characteristic is that the gold standard and the target test must measure the same characteristic or attribute.

Criterion related validity is usually established through the following procedures:

"Concurrent Validity". This is when both the target test and gold standard are given to the subjects at the same time. Those who score high in one should score high on the other. It is used mostly for situations in which the target test is either cheaper, safer, or more practical. For example using an X-ray versus a measuring tape for measuring leg length.

"Predictive Validity". This is a future-oriented type of validity where predictions are based on a measurement made today. If a subject scores well on one test, she/he will probably score well on another test.

The relationship between the target and criterion scores is examined to determine if the first test scores are predictive of the outcome on the criterion measure. For example, a researcher may be interested in knowing whether GPA in high school is predictive of high scores on the SATs. She/he may choose a group of students who are taking the SAT's and compare their scores with their high school GPA. If those who have high GPA also have high SAT scores, then the researcher establishes the predictive validity of the GPA.

4. "Construct Validity". Sometimes the variable under investigation is a construct and the researcher must establish its construct validity. Construct validity is the ability of a test to measure an abstract concept and the degree to which the test reflects the theoretical components of the concept. It is used for measuring hypothetical constructs such as intelligence, quality of life, function, endurance, fatigue, etc. This is one of the hardest types of validity to establish, as you cannot see the construct and it is not directly observable. Constructs are multidimensional, and it is hard to find out if an instrument is actually measuring all the dimensions. For example, "health" is a construct and has multiple dimensions. Therefore, it is always debatable as to how to measure "health". Are we measuring physical health, social health, cognitive health, or mental health? Therefore, for a researcher to validate an instrument that can measure multiple dimensions of health will be a challenge. Some of the ways that a construct could be validated are:

a) Known Group Method. In this process, a criterion is chosen that can identify the presence or absence of a particular characteristic and the theoretical context behind the construct is used to predict how different groups are expected to behave. For example, if a researcher wants to validate a test that measures learning disability in children, when this test is given to two groups of children, one with and one without the learning disability, their scores must be completely different so they can be differentiated from each other.

b) Multitrait - Multimethod Matrix. This test determines what a test does measure as well as what it does not measure. It is based on the concepts of ***convergent validity*** (when two tests measure the same thing) and ***discriminate validity*** (when two tests measure different things). For example, two tests that are supposed to measure the construct of "health status", when given to the same group of subjects, must produce the same results (convergent).

On the other hand, a test that measures health status and a test that is supposed to measure intelligence should not produce the same results since they are measuring two different constructs (discriminate validity).

c) Factor Analysis. Factor analysis is based on the idea that a construct holds one or more key dimensions. For example, intelligence has been analyzed in terms of memory, quantification, word fluency, perception, etc. With each of these dimensions you find a variety of tasks or performance variables that together will provide an evaluation of that particular dimension. A valid test of intelligence should be able to measure and discriminate among these components.

SUMMARY

➢ Measurement tools are invaluable in summarizing study data.
➢ Rules of measurement must be followed in order to ensure the accuracy of data collection.
➢ Awareness of the sources of measurement error allow you to construct and plan approaches to avoid them.
➢ If your tests or measurements are neither reliable nor valid, your results are ineffective.

EXERCISES FOR CHAPTERS 11-13

1- Identify the usual level of measurement for each of the following:

Year in college
Sadness
Quality of life score
Life expectancy
Endurance
Grade point average
Race
Type of society
Temperature
Pain
Height

2- What is a reliable instrument? What is a valid instrument?

3- A professor wants to give a valid test to his students to test their knowledge on the subject that he is teaching. Would you recommend one short multiple-choice test or one short essay? Why?

4- Is it possible for a test with high reliability to have low validity? Give an example.

5- A question in a questionnaire asks the respondents to identify their "family income" by choosing one of the following options:

A. $0 to $9,999
B. $10,000 to 19,999
C. $20,000 to 29,999
D. $30,000 to 39,999
E. $40,000 or 49,999
F. $50,000 or higher

What level of measurement is the researcher using to measure "family income"?

QUESTIONS FOR DISCUSSION

1- In a research report, a regular smoker is defined as "the number of times each subject said 'yes' to questions such as 'do you like smoking?' Is this definition completely operational? If not, what is missing from the definition?

2- Give an example of a gold standard measure and a related target test in your discipline. Explain how you would test the validity?

FOR STUDENTS WHO ARE PLANNING THEIR RESEARCH:

1- Define the variables that you will be studying. What level of measurement you will be using? What kinds of reliability and validity are most appropriate and explain why?

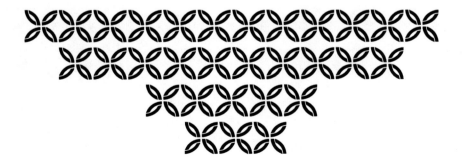

NOTES

PART V

DATA ANALYSIS

CHAPTER (14)   Descriptive Statistics
CHAPTER (15)   Correlation Statistics
CHAPTER (16)   Inferential Statistics

CHAPTER

14

DESCRIPTIVE STATISTICS

OVERALL OBJECTIVE

Develop an understanding of the role of descriptive statistics in summarizing and interpreting data.

GOALS

1. General description of different types of statistical analysis
2. Discuss ways the data could be summarized using descriptive statistics
3. Differentiate between different measures of central tendency
4. Cite the role of coefficient variations and z scores in descriptive statistics

STATISTICS

Data collected for research is in an unrefined form; it is nothing more than a bunch of numbers representing observations from groups of individuals. Statistics are rules of how to organize, summarize, and analyze your raw numbers so that they make sense and their meaning can be communicated. Without statistics, you may look at your data and make an educated guess; you may even say that there is a difference. However, there is a difference between clinical significance, and something that is statistically significant.

There are three basic fields that make up the area of statistics: *descriptive statistics, correlation statistics, and inferential statistics.*

I. Descriptive Statistics. This type of statistics, organizes the data based on two categories: measures of central tendency that include mean, median, and mode, and measures of dispersion that include standard deviation and variance.

II. Correlation Statistics. Correlation statistics, organizes and analyzes the data looking at the relationships. It can be looking for a relationship in one variable (univariate analysis), two variables (bivariate analysis) or more than two variables (multivariate analysis).

III. Inferential Statistics. Analyzes the data for two purposes: testing for the difference between the means and testing for statistical significance. The test for statistical significance has two subdivisions: parametric (when you are inferring to a large population) and non-parametric (when you are inferring to your small sample).

To Summarize:

1. Descriptive statistics (mean, median, mode; standard deviation, variance)
2. Correlation statistics (correlation, multiple correlation, and regression)
3. Inferential statistics (tests for difference of means (Z-tests), and tests for statistical significance)

TYPES OF DESCRIPTIVE STATISTICS

Descriptive statistics are used to describe the shape, central tendency, and variability in data in order to describe the population. A *parameter* is the measure of population characteristics and cannot be measured directly. Sample characteristics are called *statistics*. Researchers usually generalize the sample characteristics to the population using statistics and estimate population characteristics called *parameters*. Most researchers use descriptive statistics to look at the normality of the data. For example, descriptive analysis of age, height, sex, race, social class, level of education, etc.

Descriptive statistics summarize the data in the following forms:

A. Frequency Distribution
B. Central Tendency
C. Measures of Variability
D. Coefficient of Variation
E. Z-Score
F. Standard Error of the Mean

A. Frequency Distributions

Frequency distribution, rank orders the scores to show the number of times each value occurred, or its frequency (f). In statistics, the symbol Σ means the sum of numbers.

Σf = n (number of occurrences)

For example, the table below is the measurement of the weight (in pounds) of a group of 52 people. Data can be expressed as:

Percentage. For example, 7.6% of a sample weighs 120 *lbs*. Percentages are useful in describing distributions because they are independent of sample size, allowing for comparisons between samples of unequal size.

Cumulative Percentage. Cumulative percentage adds percentages so you may say what percentage of the entire population is below or above some number.

For example, in our group, 51.7% of the population weighs 150 pounds or less. Note that the total of individual percentages and cumulative percentages are always equal to 100%.

Table 1. Distribution of Weight of a Group of Subjects

Weight	Frequency (f)	%	Cumulative %
90	1	2	2
100	2	3.8	5.8
110	3	5.7	11.5
120	4	7.6	19.1
130	3	5.7	24.8
140	5	9.6	34.4
150	9	17.3	51.7
160	8	15.3	67
170	7	13.4	80.4
180	4	7.6	88
190	4	7.6	95.6
200	2	3.8	100
	Total		
	52	100%	

Grouped Frequency. This is for situations when every score has a frequency of one. Therefore, using a frequency distribution does not make sense anymore. The group frequency groups the scores into equal intervals and then calculates the frequency of each interval/group. For example, table 2 depicts the test scores of a group of 30 students. As you see, the frequency of every score is one. So, you can use frequency intervals of ten (40-49, 50-59, 60-69, 70-79, 80-89, 90-99 and so on). For instance, in the example below, five students fall between the intervals of 90-99 (table 3).

Table 2. Distribution of Test Score of a Group of Students

Row scores & group frequency

64	98	94	95	70	65
48	76	112	73	66	92
105	40	85	60	88	71
52	82	55	75	57	110
75	72	74	90	80	62

Table 3. Group Frequency of the Distribution of Test Score of a Group of Students

Class	Frequency
40-49	2
50-59	3
60-69	5
70-79	8
80-89	4
90-99	5
100-109	1
110-119	2

n=30

FREQUENCY DISTRIBUTION GRAPHS

Histogram
This is a bar graph, composed of a series of columns, each representing one score or class interval. The histogram for data in table 1 is as follows:

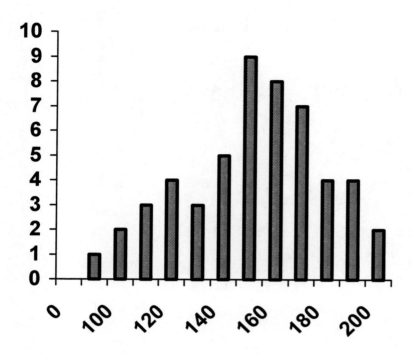

Frequency Polygon

This is a variation of the histogram in which the vertical bars are replaced by dots that are connected to form a line graph. The frequency polygon for data on table 1 is as follows:

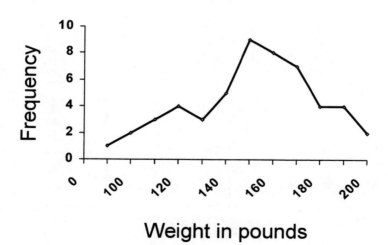

Frequency Polygon for Weights

Shapes of Distributions

Normal Distribution. Representing the data in a frequency polygon allows us to look at the shape of the distribution. In statistics a *"normal distribution"* refers to a particular bell shaped distribution, where most of the data falls in the middle and gradually less and less falls at the extremes. Each half is the mirror image of the other half. Usually, a normal curve is representative of a norm in the population. For example, if you measure the weight of the entire population, the frequency polygon would approach a normal or bell shaped curve.

"Normal" or "Bell Shaped" Curve

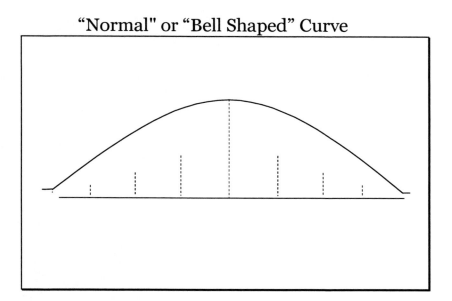

Skewed Distribution. Sometimes when you present the data on a frequency distribution graph, the graph's shape is asymmetrical. In asymmetrical distributions, the degree to which the distribution is divergent from being symmetrical is called its *skewness*. An asymmetrical distribution could be skewed to either the right or left. In *positively skewed,* or skewed to the right, distributions most of the data is clustered at the low end with only a few at the high end. This will cause the tail of the curve to point toward the right. For example, if we plot the distribution of housing prices, it will be positively skewed, because most of the houses are in a moderate to low-price range and only a few will be on the high end of the distribution. In a *negatively skewed,* or skewed to the left, distribution, most of the data is clustered at the high end of the curve and the curve points to the left. For example, a plot of the grades from an easy exam in a class could be negatively skewed; meaning that majority of the students will have a good grade and will be in the high end of the distribution.

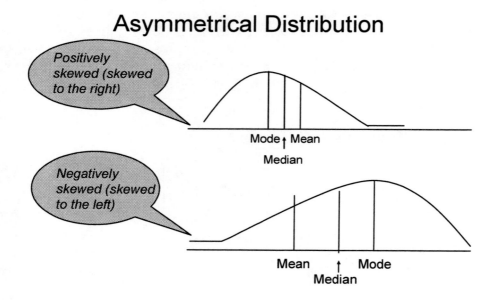

Asymmetrical Distribution

MEASURES OF CENTRAL TENDENCY

The frequency distribution allows us to understand the pattern and order of the data; however, it does not give us any numeral indices for the "norm" or "typical" nature of the data. Measures of central tendency, or averages, are numbers that describe the "*typical*" nature of the data. Where do the values tend to center? Measures of central tendency are determined in three different ways: the mode, the median, and the mean.

Mode. The mode is the most common number in a data set. The best way to find out the mode is to examine the frequency distribution and find the most frequently occurring score or number. A distribution may be bimodal (two modes) or multi-modal (more than two modes). Sometimes a distribution may not have a mode at all.

Median. The median is the middle number in the distribution when the entire data set is listed in order from low to high. Half of the numbers in the distribution fall above and half fall below the median. When the number of scores in the distribution is even, the median is the midpoint between the two numbers (calculated by adding the two middle numbers and dividing that number by two). For example, in the distribution of 3, 4, 5, 6, 7, the median is 5. In the distribution of 3, 4, 5, 6, 7, 8, the median is 5.5 (5+6/2).

Mean. The mean is the sum of all scores in the distribution divided by the total number of observations in the distribution (X= ΣX/n). The symbol use to represent the mean of the population is the Greek word mu (μ), and the bar on the top of the X represents the mean in the sample. The absolute magnitude of the data affects the mean.

Table 4 shows the scores of two groups of patients on quality of life scores (n=8 for each group). In this example, even though the distribution of scores are significantly different between the two groups (a, b), they have the same measures of central tendency for mean, mode, and median. Therefore, additional measures are needed to describe these two data sets and that is the measures of variability.

Table 4. Quality of Life Scores Obtained From Two groups of Patients

	Xa	Xb	
	88	75	
Mean = 93.66	90	79	Mean = 93.6
Median = 95	92	88	Median = 95
Mode = 95	95	95	Mode = 95
n = 8	95	95	n = 8
Range = 98-88 = 10	95	103	Range = 108-75 = 10
SD = 3.3	96	106	**SD = 11.12**
	98	108	

Σ **Xa=74**   **ΣXb=749**

MEASURES OF VARIABILITY

The explanation of a sample is not complete unless we discuss the variability that exists among the scores in the sample and its relationship with the measures of central tendency. The spread of data points around the mean is called variability. Variability in a data set could be calculated in three different ways:

1- *Range*
2- *Variance*
3- *Standard Deviation*

Range (Simplest measure of variability). Range is the difference between the maximum (highest) and the minimum (lowest) numbers in a data set. However, range does not show the difference between individual scores and is not a complete representation of variability in a data set.

Variance. Variability is the deviation of each score from the mean and the mean of these deviations is called the variance. However, because half of the data is always located above the mean and half is located below the mean, the sum of these numbers will always be zero and the mean of these numbers will be zero. To get rid of negative numbers, statisticians square all these differences and measure the sum of squared differences from the mean called the *Sum of Squares or (SS)*. When you divide the *SS* by the number of data points, you will get the mean of the squared deviation or the *Variance*. The variance for a sample is s^2 and is equal to (SS/n-1), where, SS= Σ (X-X)^2. For the population data, the symbol for variance is δ^2 and is calculated by the SS of the population divided by N (capital **N** always represents the number of data points in the population or parameter, while the small **n** represents the number of data points in the sample). Therefore, δ^2 is equal to SS/N for the population, and SS= $\Sigma(X-\mu)^2$/N.

Standard Deviation (most common). The variance is representative of variability in the sample in terms of squared units. It would be hard to explain the variability in terms of squared units such as meters squared, or pounds squared. Therefore, to bring the index of variability back to its original unit, we take the square root of the variance and call it the *standard deviation*. Standard deviation (SD) is always reported with the mean so that the data is characterized according to both the central tendency and variability. The standard deviation for a sample is calculated as (SD= $\sqrt{ss/n-1}$) and for the population the standard deviation is denoted by δ= $\sqrt{SS/N}$.

Table 5. Calculation of Some of Square and Variance

X	$X - \overline{X}$	$(X-\overline{X})^2$
1. 88	-5.6	31.36
2. 90	-3.6	12.96
3. 92	-1.6	2.5
4. 95	1.4	1.96
5. 95	1.4	1.96
6. 95	1.4	1.96
7. 96	2.4	5.75
8. 98	4.4	19.36
Σ X=749 $\overline{X}$= 93.6 n=8	$\Sigma(X-\overline{X})$= 0	SS= Σ (X- $\overline{X}$)^2= 77.81

For example, on the data sets in the previous table the calculations of variance, SD for the first column is as follow:

Variance$=S^2=$ SS/n-1 or Σ (X- $\overline{X}$)^2/n-1=
77.81/7=11.11
Standard Deviation = SD = $\sqrt{S^2}$ = $\sqrt{11.11}$=3.3

$\overline{X}$= 93.6$\pm$3.3

Coefficient of Variation (CV).
Coefficient of Variation is a measure of variability that expresses the size of the SD relative to the mean as a percentage. This is another measure of variability and is used to describe data measured on interval or ratio scales. The advantage of CV is that it is independent of units of measurement because the units will mathematically cancel out. It expresses the SD as a proportion of the mean, accounting for differences in magnitude of the mean. This is most meaningful when comparing distributions recorded in two different units. It compares the difference in the magnitudes of the means. For example, the calculation of CV for our two groups in table 4 is as follows:

CVa = SD/$\overline{X}$ * 100
3.3/93.6*100 = 3.5%

CVb = 11.12/93.6 *100 = 11.8%

This shows that the first data set is more homogenous than the second group. If you had only looked at the means of the two distributions for comparisons between these groups, it would have been appeared that there was no difference between them.

Standardized Scores (z scores).
The Z scores, expresses scores in terms of standard deviation units and are mostly used to demonstrate that an individual's score is above or below the "norm" according to the normal distribution or the normal curve. If we graph the population distribution of a variable such as height, the curve would look bell shaped with half the data recorded below the mean and the other half above the mean. In the real world, it is impossible to graph the population data; therefore, we presume that if our sample is representative of the real world, the distribution of the data should follow as closely as possible the shape of a normal curve.

Characteristics of Normal Curve
1- Mean, median, and mode are the same.
2- The data is distributed evenly on both sides of the curve, with the majority clustered around the mean.
3- 68% of the data are within $\pm$1 SD, 95% are within $\pm$2 (1.96) SD, and 99% are within $\pm$3 (2.57) SD.

The following graph represents the normal curve and the proportions of the data under the curve in regards to the standard deviations of the mean.

128

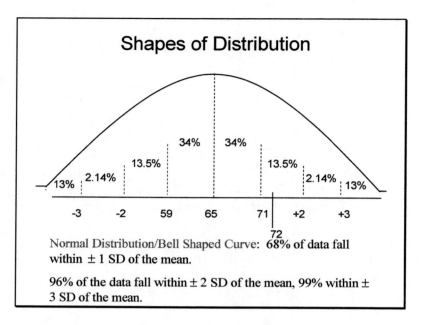

Normal Distribution/Bell Shaped Curve: 68% of data fall within ± 1 SD of the mean.

96% of the data fall within ± 2 SD of the mean, 99% within ± 3 SD of the mean.

Calculation of the Standardized Score = Z. For example, if you measure the heart rate of ten subjects and find the mean of the data is to be 65 and the SD to be 6. If you want to know the position of the subject with a heart rate of 72 within this distribution, you can calculate the Z score for this data point as follows:

Z= X-$\overline{X}$/SD

Example:

$\overline{X}$=65
SD= 6
X= 72
Z=72-65/6= 1.1

The raw score 72 is 1.1 SD above the mean. If you look at the statistical table for Z scores, you can find that the area between 0 (where the mean is) and the Z score of 1.1 is .36. If you add this to 50% of the data (data on the other half of the curve), you can say that almost 86% (50%+36%=86%) of the data is below the heart rate of 72.

Standard Error of the Mean. Standard deviation of a theoretical sampling distribution of the means is called Standard Error and is symbolized by SE. If you randomly select many samples from a population and get the mean for each sample, the mean of these sample means is considered the closest estimation of the population mean. The more samples you draw from the population and the more means you calculate, the closer you would get to the population mean. To calculate the SE from one sample, you may divide SD by the square root of the n. The idea behind this calculation is that the SD of the population is always smaller than the SD of a sample. The larger and the more homogeneous a sample, the more the sample distribution approaches the normal curve.

Standard deviation of the sampling distribution is an indicator of the degree of sampling error, reflecting how accurately various sample means estimate the population mean.
The smaller the SE, the less the scores are spread out around the mean
(SE=SD/ √ n).

SUMMARY

1- Descriptive Statistics summarizes the data in two ways:
   a. Central tendency (what is the average?)
          mean, mode, median
   b. *Variability or dispersion (how far from the average are the scores spread?)* range, variance, standard deviation

3. The measurement of Central Tendency for:
       Nominal data is mode
       Ordinal data is median
       Metric data is mean

4. The spread of variability is the *range* for nominal and ordinal data; and *variance and standard deviation* for metric data.

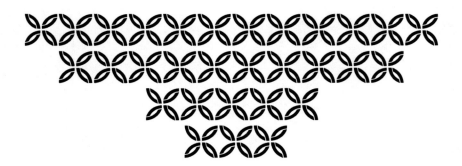

NOTES

CHAPTER

15

CORRELATION STATISTICS

OVERALL OBJECTIVE

Develop an understanding of the role of correlation statistics in analyzing and interpreting data

Goals

1. Describe correlation analyses
2. Differentiate between different types of relationships that could be established using correlation
3. Understand the application of correlation coefficient and coefficient of determination
4. Understand regression analysis and its application

CORRELATION STATISTICS

Correlation statistics are the most commonly used statistics to establish a relationship between two or more variables. *Univariate analysis* is the study of one variable for a sample, for example the age of the subjects and the analysis is often descriptive. *Bivariate analysis* is the study of a relationship between two variables; for example intensity of exercise and heart rate, and the statistical analysis is simple correlation. *Multivariate analysis* is the study of the relationship between three or more variables, for example, heart rate, intensity of exercise, and age, and the statistical analysis is multiple correlations.

Correlation Coefficient. Correlation statistics measure the strength of a relationship between two or more variables and is represented by r or the correlation coefficient. The r ranges from (+1 to −1). Note that correlation does not establish causality, but simply determines if the variables share something in common and have some relationship. In many cases there might be a third factor that causes the other two variables to change. The more two things have something in common, the more strongly they are related. The relationship could be positive (when one variable increases the other also increases) or it could be negative (when one variable increases, the other decreases). The strength of the correlation is not in the sign but in the quantity. Therefore, for correlations of −1 and +1, the strength of the correlation is high, one positively and one negatively. For example, a correlation of (-0.60) is stronger than a correlation of (+0.33).

The following table lists the interpretations for various correlation coefficients:

r = 0.8-1 --→ Strong Correlation
r= 0.6-0.7 --→Moderate Correlation
r = 0.3-0.5 --→ Weak Correlation
r = 0.0-0.2 --→Very Weak Correlation

STATISTICAL APPROACH FOR CORRELATION COEFFICIENTS

a) *Pearson's Product Moment Coefficient of Correlation.* Pearson's r is utilized with interval or ratio levels of measurements. The assumption is that the variables follow a normal distribution.

b) *Spearman's Rho Coefficient of Correlation.* The Spearman's Rho is utilized with ordinal or nominal levels of measurements, when you can rank-order your data. For example, surveys and scales.

c) *Biserial and Point Biserial Correlation.* Use biserial and point biserial approaches to examine the relationship between a continuous variable and a dichotomous attribute variable.

d) *Other techniques include*: Cronbach's coefficient (a) is used for dichotomous or discrete data and a (κ) coefficient is used for ordinal data. Depending on the level of measurement, statistical packages can be used to see if there is a significant correlation between any two variables.

APPLICATIONS OF CORRELATION

1. Prediction. Correlation could be used to predict the behavior of two related variables. For example, if you find a strong correlation between two variables (when one goes up the other also goes up), you may be able to use the performance of one variable to predict the performance of the other.

2. Measuring Consistency. In reliability testing, correlation is used to establish the reliability. For example, if the correlation between two testers' rating of

patients' performance were consistently high, this would be a good indication of their rating consistency or reliability.

3. <u>Describing Relationships.</u>   Correlation could be used to provide useful information about the relationships among variables. For example, what is the relationship between nurse supervisors' behaviors and the attitudes of nurses working under them toward patient care?

PARTIAL AND MULTIPLE CORRELATION

Partial Correlation is used to determine what correlation remains between two variables when a third variable is eliminated.

Multiple Correlation is used to find the best possible correlation between two or more variables and a dependent variable.

"CORRELATION DOES NOT MEAN CAUSATION!"

Pearson Product-Moment Correlation Coefficient
Pearson's Product-Moment Correlation Coefficient (r) represents the degree of linear *association* between any two variables. The symbol r is used for the sample data and p (*rho*) for a population. Correlation does not infer causality and it is used when two correlated variables on the X and Y-axes are continuous variables or metric level. The basic assumption behind correlation is the notion of covariance: a large y associated with a large X and a small Y is associated with a small X; X and Y co-vary, they vary in a similar pattern. Correlations are dimension-free; meaning the strength of a correlation of +1 (positive correlation) is comparable to a correlation of −1 (negative correlation). A correlation coefficient of zero, or close to zero, indicates that there is no linear relationship between the two variables.

Scatter Plots: The first step, before any correlation analysis, is to present the data on a graph, called a scatter plot. In scatter plots, each point (dot) represents the intersection of each pair of related observations. When enough data are plotted, the scatter plot could clearly show if there is a relationship between any two variables and what type of relationship there is (positive or negative).

Correlation Matrix: Researchers often examine several relationships between different variables at once. The researcher then presents all the inter-correlations between each pair of variables in a correlation matrix. If the matrix is triangular, this means that the values below the diagonal would be redundant of those above the diagonal and, therefore, would be omitted. The values on the diagonal are all 1, meaning a perfect correlation of each variable with itself.

Example of a Correlation Matrix:

Variable	A	B	C	D	E
A	1.00	.003	.13	.89*	.97*
B		1.00	.45*	.12	.111
C			1.00	.16	.55*
D				1.00	.92*
E					1.00

As you can see, the correlation of each variable with itself is 1.00 and the asterisks are indications of significant correlation.

Application of Hypothesis Testing for Correlation Analysis

Step 1: H_0: p or $r = 0$

   H_1: $p > 0$ or H_1: $r > 0$

Step 2: alpha = 0.05

Step 3: Determine the appropriate statistics: Pearson r, Spearman rank order, etc.

Step 4: Determine the critical statistical value (df = n-2)

Step 5: Calculate the statistic r or p values and compare with the critical value to determine significance.

Coefficient of Determination (CD) (r^2)

One should be careful not to interpret the correlation coefficient in terms of percentages. For example, a correlation of 0.80 does not mean that when one variable varies, the other variable varies 80 percent of the time. For this type of information, researchers use another determination called the coefficient of determination, which means when one factor varies, the other varies a specific percentage of the time. The coefficient of determination is the square of the correlation coefficient.

Example: if $r = .80$
      $r^2 = 64\%$

The percentage of change of one variable in relation to another variable is 64 percent of the time. The coefficient of determination is the measure of variance shared by, or common to, two variables. It shows the strength of the correlation (r^2 x 100). The significant r only means that the relationship really exists, but it does not say how strong it is. As sample size increases, even a weak correlation of 0.2 may show significance. When CD= 4% (r^2), it means that only 4% of the variability is shared by the two variables, which is not very strong.

REGRESSION ANALYSIS

One of the most popular methods of conducting an analysis of the relationship between two or more variables is building a linear regression equation. The regression model is based on correlation, if the variable of interest is correlated with the other variable(s) under investigation in the study, then one can assume that the estimated equation will be able to accurately predict the response variable. The linear regression equation is used to explain or predict the variable of interest based on the changes in the function of other variables. On one side of the regression equation is the variable of interest and on the other side of the equation is the linear function of the other variable(s). Using sample data, this analysis allows us to estimate the parameters (slope and intercepts of the regression equation). After building the regression model, it should be tested using empirical data from the sample to evaluate the predictive power of the equation. Most statistical computer packages can help you develop an accurate regression model, given a dataset with correlated data fields.

Regression Line. The single straight line that is placed closest to all of the points in a scatter plot is called a regression line. The regression line can be used for making correlation predictions when three important pieces of information are known: 1) how much the scatter points deviate from the line, 2) the slope of the line, and 3) the point of intercept.

$Y = a + b X$
Y = predicted score or dependant variable
X = score for the independent variable
b = slope of the regression line, the regression coefficient represents the change in y for each one unit change in x
a = y intercept, regression constant, represents the value of y when x = 0
a and b can be calculated based on the formulas of a known data set for X and Y.

In regression, researchers may be able to estimate the causality in data analysis. The researcher tries to predict how close the data can be "fitted" to the estimated straight line. Linear regression and the least squares method are the most common forms of regression. During these computations, a researcher attempts to find the equation that best fits a line representing what is called the regression of y (dependent variable or criterion variable) on x (independent variable or predictor variable) regardless of the scattering of the data points. The slope of the line (equation) gives information about predicted directionality and the estimated coefficients for x and y (independent and dependent variables) indicating the power of the relationship.

The regression formula creates a number called R-squared, which is like a coefficient of determination. For interpretation of R-squared, the researcher usually uses the same strength table as in correlation coefficients. When b (regression coefficient) is positive, y increases as x increases. When b is negative, y decreases as x increases.

If $b = 0$, the slope of the line is horizontal, indicating no relationship between x and y. The positive or negative direction of the slope will correspond to a positive or negative correlation between x and y. There are also advanced regression techniques for curvilinear estimation.

Multiple Regression. Sometimes a researcher may be interested in multiple regressions by making a prediction from two or more variables. Techniques using the multiple R for making predictions of one variable given measures on two or more other variables are called multiple regressions. It is more accurate than simple linear regression since more variables are used to make the prediction. It requires the calculation of the intercept (a) and at least two slopes (b_1 and b_2). For the three-variable situation, the multiple regression equation is as follows: $Y = a + b_1X + b_2X^2 + b_3X^3$

EXERCISES FOR CHAPTERS 14-15

1- Which number is the most frequently occurring score in a data set?
2- What is the relationship between the mean and standard deviation? Why is it important that they be reported together?
3- Should the mean be reported for a positively or negatively skewed distribution? Explain.
4- What is the difference between r and r^2? Explain.
5- The middle 68% of a normal distribution has scores between what two numbers, if the mean is 50 and the standard deviation is 10?
6- If the mean $\pm$ the standard deviation for two different data sets are: 65 ± 5 and 2.5 ± 1, which data set has less variability? Show your calculations.

QUESTIONS FOR DISCUSSION

1- Suppose a researcher reports his data and says "the average was 23". What additional information should you ask for? Why?
2- Name two variables for which you would expect to see a strong relationship.

FOR STUDENTS DOING THEIR RESEARCH

1- Are you going to use descriptive or correlation analysis for your research? What variables would you describe in your descriptive data analysis. If you are doing correlation, what relationships you are trying to establish? Explain.

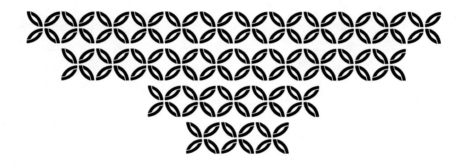

NOTES

CHAPTER

16

INFERENTIAL STATISTICS

OVERALL OBJECTIVE

To develop an understanding of various statistical tests that can guide the interpretation of the research results.

GOALS

1. Describe the characteristics of hypotheses and differentiate between null and alternative hypotheses
2. Cite the roles of significance and power
3. Discuss the factors involve in determining and increasing the power of a test
4. Differentiate between parametric and non-parametric statistics
5. Describe the steps involved in the hypothesis testing procedure
6. Illustrate how to apply the hypothesis testing procedure to parametric and non-parametric statistics.

INFERENTIAL STATISTICS

Inferential statistics, also called inductive statistics, are the strongest type of analysis. It involves the decision making process and making predictions based on a small, representative sample. Inferential statistics fall into two classes: *tests for difference of means* and *tests for statistical significance*. The test for statistical significance can be subdivided into *parametric and non-parametric statistics*. *Parametric statistics* are utilized when the researcher has a large representative sample and is inferring the results to the larger population as a whole. *Non-parametric statistics* are used when the sample is small and the researcher uses the results to make inferences only to the people in the sample.

The most common technique for testing statistical difference of the means is the Z -test. The most common parametric statistics are the t-test, F-test, ANOVA, and regression. The most common non-parametric tests of significance are Chi-Square, the Mann-Whitney U-test, and the Kruskal-Wallis test.

Basic assumptions in inferential statistics are based on the three concepts: probability, sampling error, and confidence intervals.

Probability (p)

Probability is the proportion of time that we expect a given outcome to happen given all other possibilities, and is expressed as a ratio or a decimal and is denoted by the symbol (p). For example, the probability of a coin toss being either head or tail is 50% because there are only two possible events that may occur at any time. For a dice with 6 sides, and 6 possible occurrences, the chance of any number occurring is 1 out of 6, or $p = 0.167$. Overall, for an event that is certain to occur, $p = 1.00$, and for an impossible event, $p = 0.00$. Nothing is 100% sure of happening and nothing is "impossible". Probability in research is used to predict what should happen over the long run.

Application of Probability in Research
1. Make decisions about how well sample data estimates the characteristics of a population
2. Determine if observed treatment differences are likely to be representative of population differences or if they happen by chance
3. Estimate what would happen to others in the population on the basis of a small sample.

Sampling Error
Sampling error is the propensity for sample values to be different from population values. It is unpredictable and happens strictly by chance. As sample size increases, the sample becomes more representative of the population and their mean is more likely to be closer to the population mean; that is, their sampling error will be smaller.

Standard Error of the Mean
The standard deviation of a theoretical sampling distribution of means is called the Standard Error and is denoted by SE. If you randomly select many samples from a population and get the mean for each sample, the means of these sample means are considered the closest estimate of the population mean. The more samples you draw from the population, the more means you create, and the closer you get to the population mean. The distribution of sample means is called *sampling distribution of the means*, which consistently takes the shape of a

normal curve. It is very hard and time consuming to continuously draw samples from the population in order to calculate the population standard deviation; therefore, the standard deviation of the population (standard error of the means) is calculated from one sample by dividing that sample's standard deviation by the square root of the sample size $(SE=SD/\sqrt{n})$. The idea behind this calculation is that the SD of a population is always smaller than the SD of a sample. As sample size increases, the sample mean approaches the population mean, or the sample distribution approaches the normal curve.

Confidence Intervals (CI)

The main purpose of research is to select a representative sample from a population and estimate the characteristics of the population using that sample. There are two ways that a researcher could make this estimate:

Point estimate: This is to find out the mean for the sample and apply that as the estimate of the population mean. For example, if the mean for the sample data is 30, you would say μ (population mean) is also 30.

Confidence Interval (CI): We know that any sample that we choose from a population will have a different mean than the population mean. Confidence Interval (CI) is proposing a boundary, or range of values, within which the researcher estimates that the population mean will be located. In another words, it is the range of scores that should contain the population mean and is calculated based on the sample mean and the standard error. The confidence limits are based on a probability of either 95% or 99%. The larger the boundary, the greater the possibility that the population mean will fall within that boundary. For example, the researcher may say she/he is 95% or 99% confident that the population mean is within this boundary.

The calculation of the CI is based on the assumptions of a normal curve. If you remember, we said that 95% of the population falls between ±2 standard deviation (SD) and 99% of the population falls between ± 3 SD. To estimate the boundaries with confidence, statisticians propose values that are a little less than 2 and 3 SD. If you look at the table for values of Z scores (available in most statistical books and computer statistical packages), you see that 95% of the population falls between Z scores of ±1.96 (a little less than 2) and 99% of the population falls between Z scores of ± 2.57 (a little less than 3). The calculation of CI for 95% and 99% for any sample are as follows:

Calculation of CI for Large Sample
(95% confidence interval)

95% CI = $\overline{X} \pm$ (1.96) SE
For example, if the sample mean is 65 and SE is 3, CI will be calculated as follows:

95% CI = $65 \pm 1.96 * 3$

95% CI = 65± 5.88

95% CI = 59.12 $\leq u \leq$ 70.88
We are 95% confident that the population mean is between 61.25 and 68.75.

Calculation of 99% confidence interval:
(99% CI = $\overline{X}$ + (2.57) SE)

For *example*, if the sample mean is 65 and SE is 3, CI will be calculated as follows:

99% CI = 65 $\pm$ 2.57* 3
99% CI = 65 $\pm$ 7.71
99% CI = 57.29 $\leq u \leq$ 72.71
We are 99% confident that the population mean is between 57.29 and 72.71.

As you can see, as you increase your confidence level, the estimating boundaries also increase. In other words, the confidence limits get wider as our confidence interval increases.

CI with Small Samples
For small samples, usually less than 30, sampling distributions are likely to be more spread out than normal distributions. Therefore, the standard normal curve is not a good representation of small distributions (with samples < 30). The alternative theoretical sampling distribution, called the **"t-distribution"**, is usually used to represent the smaller samples. The **t- curve** is flatter and wider at the tails than the normal curve and changes with different sample sizes. As sample size increases, the distribution approaches the shape of the normal curve. To calculate the CI for a small sample size, the following formula is applied:

$CI = \overline{X} \pm (t) SE$
The values of *t* for confidence levels of 95% and 99% are calculated based on the *degree of freedom (df)* or *n-1* for each sample. Statistical tables for the *t distribution* have been developed and could be used to calculate the 95% and 99% CI for specific sample sizes.
(*df* = n - 1: number of components that are free to vary within a set of data and is always one less than the total sample size. For example, for a sample size of 29, the *df* is 29-1=28).

Application of Confidence Intervals
Confidence intervals in research are mostly used for establishing the "norms" for population characteristics. We can use confidence intervals to estimate normative population values and these norms can be used for the purpose of clinical decision-making. For example, a researcher may establish the normal range of motion of a joint in the body. Then clinicians may examine their patients to see if the range of motion of a specific joint is within the normal range or not.

Note** Statistical software packages easily calculate the CI as part of the descriptive analysis of the data.

HYPOTHESES

A. Definition. Hypotheses are intelligent or educated guesses made regarding the outcome of an experiment before all the facts are recognized. In experimental and correlational research, the researcher normally tests the hypotheses by designing an experiment and collecting and analyzing data in order to provide proof so that the hypothesis could be accepted or rejected.

B. Characteristics of Hypotheses. Hypotheses are statements that predict relationships between the IV and the DV in a population. They usually incorporate phrases such as "greater than" or "less than", to indicate types of relationships. The most important characteristics of a hypothesis are that it has to be testable, acceptable, and based on sound rationale. A hypothesis can be either "deductive" or "inductive".

C. Alternate/Research Hypothesis (HA). It is an if-then statement, an intelligent guess about the nature of an answer to a question. An alternative hypothesis is always stated in a positive format and will be used as a guide for the interpretation of outcomes and conclusion of the study.
The alternative hypothesis could be *directional or non-directional.* A directional hypothesis is when the researcher guesses the direction of the response under investigation, or which "mean" is going to be larger after an intervention. In non-directional hypotheses, the researcher is not certain about the direction of the response.

For example, a researcher randomly chooses two groups of subjects. One group (experimental) will receive an exercise intervention for three months and the other group (control) will receive no intervention. The dependant variables are heart rate and blood pressure.
The researcher may have *a directional hypothesis* stating:
The mean resting heart rate and blood pressure of the experimental group will be lower than the control group after three months of an exercise intervention.

....or she/he may have *a non-directional hypothesis* stating:
The mean heart rate and blood pressure of the experimental group will be different than the control group after three months of an exercise intervention.

The following is how a researcher usually describes the alternative or research hypothesis:

H1: $\mu A \neq \mu B$, or H1: $\mu A - \mu B \neq 0$ (non-directional)
H1: $\mu A > \mu B$ or H1: $\mu A < \mu B$ (directional)

D. Null/Statistical Hypothesis (H$_O$). The null hypothesis is the statistical hypothesis and states that that there is no difference or relationship among variables. It challenges the alternative hypothesis by stating that the changes are due to chance and not due to a real difference. Using statistical analysis and the rules of probability, the researcher tries to reject the null hypothesis and prove the research hypothesis. In the real world, nothing is a sure bet, therefore, you can never actually "prove" or "disprove" the null hypothesis. The purpose of an experiment is to give the data a chance to reject the false null hypothesis. The null hypothesis is always stated in a negative format and basically says that there is no relationship between the DV and IV.

Ho: $\mu A = \mu B$ or Ho: $\mu A - \mu B = 0$

HYPOTHESIS TESTING

A. Considerations
B. Testing in Research
C. Decisions
D. Level of Significance
E. Power

A. Considerations: Statistical tests either reject or fail to reject Ho. If we reject Ho, then there is a difference or relationship between the means. By rejecting the null hypothesis, we conclude that it is unlikely that chance is operating to produce observed differences, or there is strong evidence to support the research hypothesis. If we fail to reject Ho, then a difference, or a relationship, does not exist or there is not enough evidence to contradict the null hypothesis.

B. Hypothesis Testing in Research: Are based on the correct or incorrect decisions that you make following your research. The following diagram shows all the possible decisions when testing a hypothesis.

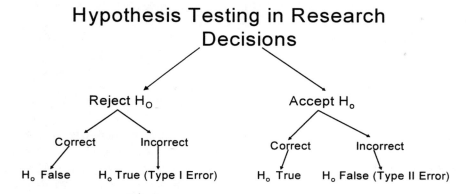

Hypothesis Testing in Research Decisions

Correct Decision: Accepting H_O when it is true and
Rejecting H_O when it is false

C. Decisions: The decision to reject or not to reject the null hypothesis is based on the results, accurate statistical testing, and representativeness of the sample data. It is always possible that even with the most proper statistical testing, we may make a wrong decision. Therefore, the process of hypothesis testing will always result in two types of decisions, either to reject or fail to reject the null hypothesis. Either one of these decisions may be right or wrong. The wrong decisions are considered either Type I or Type II errors.

Type I error (alpha, α)
Type I error is rejecting H_o when it is true. The researcher concludes that a true difference exists between population means, when differences are due to chance.

Type II error (beta, β)
Type II error is accepting H_o when it is false. The researcher concludes that the differences are due to chance when it is a true difference in population means.

The seriousness of one type of error over the other is relative; however, most researchers focus on Type I error as the primary basis for hypothesis testing.

D. Level of significance: The level of significance is the chance, or risk that a researcher is willing to take, of being wrong when rejecting the H_o. This is a standard to determine the probability of committing a Type I error for rejecting the null hypothesis. It represents a standard for decision making as to whether the differences are due to chance, sampling error, or are due to real differences. The larger the observed difference, the less likely it occurred by chance.
The maximum acceptable risk of making a Type I error if we reject H_o is denoted as the *level of significance or α.* Typically, we set α at 0.05, which is considered a very small risk. We are willing to accept a 5% chance of incorrectly rejecting H_o.
Remember that, α. = .05 does not mean that there is a 95% chance that the alternative hypothesis is true.

Type II error or β means that we do not reject the null hypothesis when it is indeed false or we find no significant difference when a difference really exists. It is denoted by β, or Type II error, and is usually set at 0.20, meaning that we are willing to accept a 20% chance of failing to reject the false null hypothesis.

E. Statistical Power = 1-β: The power of statistical analysis is the probability that a test will lead to the rejection of the null hypothesis and is denoted as (1 - 0.20 = 0.80). There is an 80% chance/probability of correctly showing statistical differences and rejecting H_o if actual differences exist. The more powerful a statistical test is, the less likely it is of making a Type II error. The power of a test depends on the level of significance, sample size, and the effect size. Effect size index is obtained by substituting values for sample means and standard deviation; the larger the effect size is, the more powerful the test will be. The effect size is estimated based on clinical experience, pilot data, or previous research that examined the same variables. The larger the sample size and the effect size, the higher the probability that a test may find a significant difference.

Probabilities of Being Correct or Incorrect

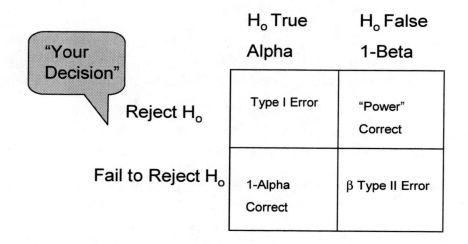

Power Analysis

Power analysis is a statistical procedure used to estimate the level of power required to reject the false null hypothesis in a particular study. Most researchers carry out a power analysis before they start their study to estimate the sample size they need to show significance.

Purposes of Power Analysis in Research

1. Power analysis in research is used to estimate the sample size needed before data collection. By specifying the level of significance and desired power in the early planning stages of a study, you can estimate how many subjects would be needed to detect significant differences. This is done prospectively before the study starts.

2. The researcher may use power analysis retrospectively to determine the probability that a Type II error was committed with non-significant findings. By knowing the level of significance, variance, sample size and effect size, if the power was low, the researcher may conclude that the results should be evaluated with caution and propose to replicate the study with more subjects. This is done retrospectively after the study is completed.

Statistical Power of a test is a function of four criterions:
1. Significance level (α)
2. Variance (s^2)
3. Sample size (n)
4. Effect size (ES)

1. Significance level (α)

This is the probability of correctly rejecting a false H_o. The researcher should minimize alpha and beta, and maximize 1-alpha and 1-beta (power). Usually α is pre-set at 0.05, $(p \leq 0.05)$. This means that the researcher is willing to allow a 5% chance of making a Type I error and falsely rejecting the null hypothesis when the null is actually correct. β is usually pre-set at 0.20, meaning that the researcher is willing to allow a 20% chance of making a Type II error and wrongfully accepting the null hypothesis when the null is actually wrong. 1-β, or (1-0.20 = 0.80), is considered the power of the statistical analysis; meaning that with the alpha level of 0.05, and beta at 0.20, there is an 80% chance that this analysis will be detecting a true difference. Usually researchers determine the relative risks of making Type I & II errors, and pre-set the alpha & beta accordingly.

2. Variance

The power of a statistical test will increase as the variance within a set of data decreases, or when the data is more homogeneous. Large variability within a group will reduce the detection of true differences between groups.

3. Sample size

The larger the sample size, the greater the power will be. Small samples are not good representations of a population. However, the most important point in sample size determination is that the sample must be a good representation of the population under investigation. The more diverse the population, the larger the sample size should be.

4. Effect Size (ES)

Effect size is the difference between the mean responses of your experimental and control groups. It is the measure of the magnitude of differences between sample means expressed in standard deviation (SD) units. The larger the difference is, the higher the chance of rejecting the null hypothesis will be (higher power).

Small effect size: Small ES = 0.2 (the difference between means is approximately 20% of the group SD). This is when changes are not perceivable to the human eye, but not so small as to be minute; or when a phenomenon under study is not well understood.

Medium effect size: Medium ES = 0.5 (the difference between means is approximately 50% of the group SD). When changes are either large enough to be visible to the naked eye, or one could be aware of the changes in the course of normal observation.

Large effect size: Large ES = 0.8 (the difference between means is approximately 80% of the group SD). There is a great degree of separation, so that there is very little overlap between population distributions. Differences should be grossly observable.

Power can be determined based on the investigator's knowledge of the estimated ES (means, SDs), sample size, and alpha level. The investigator must have good prior knowledge to estimate ES. In order to find the most appropriate effect size, it is best to find other researchers' data (mean ± SD, correlation) for similar experiments and use the same level of expected effect size. Sometimes an investigator may perform a small study with a small sample as a pilot and estimate effect size from that. If ES cannot be estimated the following table could be used to estimate the necessary sample sizes for a given level of power and effect size (alpha = .05).

Simple Power Table

Necessary Sample Sizes for each group at given levels of power & effect size (alpha = .05).

Effect size	Power 0.5	0.7	0.9
− 0.2 (very small)	195	325	>500
− 0.4 (small)	50	78	132
− 0.6 (medium)	22	36	58
− 0.8 (large)	13	21	34
− 1.0 (very large)	8	11	22
− 1.5 (giant)	4	6	11

Practical recommendations for power analysis and sample size determination:

1- For a given sample size, a large ES is necessary to achieve high power.

2- For a given level of power, the smaller the ES, the larger the sample size needed to attain statistical significance.

3- The smaller the ES, the larger the sample size needed to attain statistical significance.

4- Plan your study: Find out about all the aspects of your study including the:

➢ Sample size available
➢ Expected variability
➢ Desired ES
➢ Relative importance of Type I & II errors

5- To increase power:

➢ Perform a priori power analysis
➢ Increase sample size
➢ Increase homogeneity
➢ Remove extraneous variability
➢ Increase precision & accuracy of testing instruments
➢ Increase effect size
➢ Look for big, clinically significant differences

PARAMETRIC STATISTICS *metric / (interval – ratio scale)*

Parametric statistics are used to estimate population parameters from a sample and require several specific conditions/assumptions that the data must meet before analysis. Parametric statistics are used mostly with metric (interval and ratio) data and can be subjected to arithmetic manipulations (Mean, SD). They are more statistically powerful than non-parametric statistics. When their application is justified, parametric statistics are preferred because they are more powerful and more versatile with complex research designs. The most common parametric tests of significance are the F-test, t-test, ANOVA, and regression.

NON-PARAMETRIC STATISTICS *(nominal – ordinal data)*

Non-parametric statistics require fewer assumptions and are used with nominal and ordinal data. They are less statistically powerful because most of them involve ranking scores rather than comparing precise metric changes. Non-parametric statistics are most useful when ordinal or nominal data are collected and when samples are small and normality cannot be assumed. The most common non-parametric tests of significance are chi-square, the Mann-Whitney U-test, and the Kruskal-Wallis test.

Steps in Data Analysis Techniques

1. Identify the population to which the findings of the research are applied
2. State the research hypothesis

3.   Select the sample from the population using random sampling
4.   Conduct the research study on the sample
5.   Infer the results of the study to the population

Hypothesis-Testing Procedure

Researchers use a 5-step procedure to decide whether to accept or reject the research hypothesis based on the information collected on the sample(s) in the research study.

Step 1: State the Hypothesis

H_0: $\mu_1 = \mu_2$ (null hypothesis or no difference)
H_1: $\mu_1 > \mu_2$ or $\mu_1 < \mu_2$ ------> Directional
H_1: $\mu_1 \neq \mu_2$ ------> Non-Directional

Step 2: Select the significance Level

The difference between the population mean and what is found in the sample is either due to the null hypothesis being false or due to sampling error. To answer the research question, the researcher performs a statistical test to find out the probability that the difference is due to chance or to actual differences. The level of significance is the maximum risk that a researcher is willing to take in order to accept that the differences are due to chance and is usually set at $\alpha = 0.05$.

Step 3: Consult the Appropriate Statistical Table

If you remember from the section on confidence intervals, 95% of the data lies between the Z scores of $\pm$ 1.96 and only 5% lies on the other two sides of the curve. When you choose a sample and introduce an intervention, you would expect that after the intervention this sample mean would be different from the sample mean before the intervention. In other words, due to the intervention your sample has changed and now represents a different population. If you compare the distribution of these two samples, you would expect two different curves with different means and standard deviations. For each data set, you are 95% confident that the population means for each data sets lies between the Z scores of $\pm$ 1.96 relative to their related standard error. Therefore, there is only a 5% chance that the population means for these two data sets are the same. The area between the Z scores of $\pm$ 1.96 is considered the **critical region** and the value of Z that defines this area is called the **critical value**. However, because nothing is a sure bet, you are willing to accept some possibility that the two samples are the same. The level of significance of .05 indicates that you are willing to accept that there is a 5% chance that the two populations that are represented by these samples are the same.

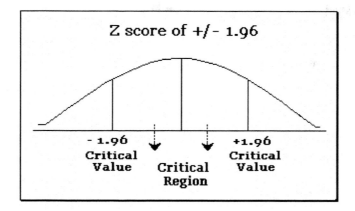

Most researchers examine an appropriate statistical table to find the value that the statistical test of the sample would need to be equal or exceed in order to reject the null hypothesis at the specific alpha level. Many computer programs provide a probability value (p) for the value of the statistical test selected. The researcher rejects the null if the *p* value is equal or less than the alpha values (usually set at $\alpha = 0.05$).

Step 4: Tests for Statistical Significance

To test for statistical significance the researcher:
First, randomly assigns the sample to two independent groups. The null hypothesis assumes the sample means are the same and that the individual differences are evenly distributed among groups.
After the application of some independent variable, the researcher evaluates the sample means for significant differences through a test of statistical significance by calculating the statistical ratio. The larger the ratio, the more significant the test will be.

Statistical ratio = $\dfrac{\text{difference between group means (effect size)}}{\text{variability within groups}}$

Step 5: Accept or Reject the Null Hypothesis

This is the decision making step, in which the researcher either accepts or rejects the null hypothesis. If the value for statistical ratio is larger than the critical value, the null hypothesis will be rejected. If the opposite is true, the null hypothesis will not be rejected.

THE T-TEST

It is used to compare two means to see if there is a significant difference between them.

TYPES
1. One group paired t-test
2. Independent sample -test
3. Two groups unequal variance

1- One Group Paired t-test
This is the simplest statistical test that is used when there is a repeated measure or matched pair design. The test analyzes the difference in scores within each subject (d) or matched pairs of subjects. The ratio reflects the relationship of *between* and *within* group variances.

Calculation of t-Statistics:

$t = \bar{d}/ \bar{s_d}$

d = mean of difference in scores, and s $_d$ = standard error of difference scores, and the degree of freedom is n-1. The numerator is the difference between pairs of scores and the denominator is the variability within the difference in scores.

Application of Hypothesis Testing

Step 1: Make the assumption that there is no difference between pre and post score means (null hypothesis).

$H_o = \mu A = \mu B$
H1: $\mu A \neq \mu B$, or H1: $\mu A - \mu B = 0$ (non-directional)
H1: $\mu A > \mu B$ or H1: $\mu A < \mu B$ (directional)

Step 2: Set the α level at 0.05

Step 3: Consult the statistical t-table for a specific sample size and α level

Step 4: Calculate the mean for pre and post data
Calculate the t-test (critical statistical value)

Step 5: Take this number and compare it to the "critical value of t" in the table; if your "observed" value exceeds the critical value, then you have found a significant difference between the means.

Examples of Two Dependent Groups t-test
Repeated measures design. Pre-test / Post-test
measurement ---> treatment ---> measurement

Match Pairs Design. Subjects will be matched in pairs and then, randomly one subject will receive treatment A and one subject will receive treatment B (or no treatment).

2- T- TEST FOR INDEPENDENT SAMPLES

Unpaired t-test.   This test compares two independent groups of subjects. Groups are created through random assignment. Subjects are randomly assigned to two independent groups, an experimental and a control group. The experimental group receives the intervention and the control group is observed under controlled conditions with no intervention. The independent *t*-test helps you decide whether the observed difference between 2 sample means happened by chance or is a true difference. The independent *t*-test is based on the assumption that the variability of the scores between the two groups is equal. This is called the assumption of *equality of variance, or homogeneity of variance.* The two most common tests used to establish this equality are Levene's test and Bartlett's test. If the difference in variability of the two groups is not significant, the two groups are considered equal. Both tests are based on the F-test.

Statistical ratio for the unpaired *t*-test is calculated as follow:

$$t = \frac{\bar{X}_1 - \bar{X}_2}{S_{\bar{X}_1 - \bar{X}_2}}$$

$S_{\bar{X}_1 - \bar{X}_2}$ is the standard error of the difference between the means. It is also called the pooled variance estimate. The degrees of freedom (df) to calculate the *t* ratio is $= (n_1 + n_2) - 2$.

Application of Hypothesis Testing

Step 1: Make the assumption that there is no difference between two sample means (null hypothesis).

$H_o = \mu A = \mu B$
$H1: \mu A \neq \mu B$, or $H1: \mu A - \mu B \neq 0$ *(non-directional)*
$H1: \mu A > \mu B$ or $H1: \mu A < \mu B$ *(directional)*

Step 2: $\alpha = 0.05$

Step 3: Find the critical value in the t- table
        ($\alpha / 2$ = two tailed)

Step 4: Calculate the t-test

Step 5: Accept or reject the null hypothesis based on the value of the calculated *t* - ratio.   If the calculated *t* is larger than the critical *t*-value, the null hypothesis is rejected and you have support for your alternative hypothesis.

Sign of t

Critical values for *t* are independent of sign; therefore, the sign of *t* whether positive or negative is tested against the same criteria. The sign can also be ignored in non-directional hypothesis. The critical region for a two-tailed test (non-directional) is located in both tails of the *t* distribution curve. Therefore, both positive and negative values are considered significant. The sign of *t* is important when you are making a directional hypothesis. The researcher predicts that one mean will be larger than the other; therefore, the hypothesis must be tested against the direction that the researcher predicts. For example, if the researcher predicts that the mean for sample A will be larger than sample B, but at the conclusion of the study, he finds that the mean for sample B is larger than sample A. The hypothesis is defeated and the researcher cannot change the direction of the hypothesis. A directional hypothesis, however, is statistically more powerful in finding statistical significance since the critical region is located only on one side of the t distribution. The most important thing is that the researcher must be confident in the direction that he or she proposes.

3- T-TEST FOR UNEQUAL VARIANCE

This is for situations where there is a difference in sample size and variability between the two samples and you cannot establish equality of variance between the two groups. The t ratio used for this situation is based on separate variances of the two groups and not the pooled variance.

$$t = \frac{\overline{X_1} - \overline{X_2}}{\sqrt{\dfrac{S_1^2}{n_1} + \dfrac{S_2^2}{n_2}}}$$

ANALYSIS OF VARIANCE (ANOVA) > 2 groups

Analysis of Variance (ANOVA) is a data analysis procedure that is similar to the t-test *EXCEPT* it is used when more than 2 groups are involved. It can be applied to independent groups or repeated measures designs. ANOVA basically reveals the main and interaction effects of independent variables (IV) (called "factors") on dependent variables (DV). The "main effect" is the direct effect of an independent variable on the dependent variable. An "interaction effect" is the combined effects of two or more independent variables or levels of the independent variable(s) on the dependent variable(s). ANOVA is based on the "*F*" statistic.

$$F = \frac{\text{between-groups treatment effect}}{\text{within-groups variability}}$$

The *F*-test is used to ascertain how much of the total observed variability in scores can be explained by the differences between treatment means versus how much is caused by variability among subjects. To analyze this variability among treatment groups, the sum of squares (SS) is calculated by subtracting the sample mean from each score (X-$\overline{X}$), squaring those values, and taking their sum. The larger the sums of squares are, the larger the variability of scores within a sample. A significant *F* test shows that there is an overall effect of the independent variable on the dependant variable; however, it does not show where the relationship is. The *multiple comparison tests* of significance will then be used to explore where exactly the differences exist.

If the data involves repeated measures of the same variable, as in before-after, or matched pair tests, the *F*-test is computed differently from the usual between-groups design, but the inference logic is the same. There are also a large variety of other ANOVA designs for special purposes, all with the same logic.

One-Way ANOVA

Involves statistical analysis of 3 or more independent groups. One-way means one independent variable (IV) with 3 or more levels.

For example: What is the effect of aerobic exercise on blood pressure if it is performed once per week, twice per week, or three times per week?

Exercise = IV, once per week, twice per week and three times per week are the three levels. You would require at least three groups to make the comparison. The ANOVA will tell you if there is a difference between these groups; however, it does not tell you where the differences are. To find out where the differences are, the researcher should do another analysis called *multiple comparisons tests*.

Terms Used to Perform an ANOVA:

k = Number of independent groups

N = Total number of subjects each receiving different treatments

T = Total

W = Within

A = Among

df = degrees of freedom

SS_T = Sum of squares <u>total</u>: Is the variability of the scores from means for all the groups combined.

SS_A = Sum of squares <u>among</u> groups: Is an indication of differences among groups.

$\overline{X}$-$\overline{X}G$ (grand mean)

df_A = k (number of groups) - 1

SS_W: Sum of squares <u>within</u> groups: Is an indication of how much the scores in the groups differ from their group mean. X-$\overline{X}$,

df_W = N (total number of subjects) - k (number of groups)

- $SS_T = SS_A + SS_W$
- $df_T = df_A + df_W$
- $df_T = N - 1$

- $df_A = k - 1$
- $df_W = N - k$
- $MS_W = SS_W/df_W$
- $MS_A = SS_A/df_A$
- $MS_W = SS_W/df_W$
- $F = MS_A/MS_W$

F value has two degrees of freedom: $k - 1$ and $N - k$

The larger the calculated F values from the reported critical values for F statistics table, the higher the possibility of significance in the results.

Application of Hypothesis Testing in One Way ANOVA

Step 1: H_0: $\mu_a = \mu_b = \mu_c$

      H_1: $\mu_a \neq \mu_b \neq \mu_c$

Step 2: $\alpha = 0.05$

Step 3: Degrees of freedom

      $k - 1$ and $N - k$

Step 4: Find the F ratio

      $F = MS_A/MS_W$

Step 5: Compare the F ratio to the critical value for F Statistics.

Summary Table for a Hypothetical One-Way Analysis of Variance

N= 15, K=3

Source of Variance	DF	SS	MS	F	P
Between Groups (b)	2 (k-1)	180	115	9.86	<0.01
Error (within Groups) (w)	12 (N-K)	140	12.5		
Total	14 (N-1)	270			

(0.05) $F_{(2, 12)} = 3.89$

Two-Way ANOVA

This analysis involves two independent variables, one of which may be conceived as a control variable. It has two components of between group variance and error variance. The between group variance explains the independent variable effects, and the error variance accounts for variability in response not related to the treatments.

It tries to answer the following questions:

What is the effect of variable A, independent of variable B?

What is the effect of variable B, independent of variable A?
What is the joint effect, or interaction, of variable A and B?

Multivariate or N-way ANOVA

This analysis involves (n) independent variables (more than two). As the number of independent variables increases, the number of potential interactions also increases. Two independent variables have a single, first-order interaction (AB). Three independents have four interactions: three first order interactions (AB, AC, BC) and one second-order interaction (ABC). Four independents have ten interactions: six first-order (AB, AC, AD, BC, BC, CD), three second-order (ABC, ACD, BCD), and one third-order (ABCD) interaction. As the number of interactions increases, it becomes increasingly difficult to interpret the model.

Repeated Measures, or Within-Groups, ANOVA Design

This analysis is used when subjects are used as their own control. Either time is the repeated factor in which a dependent variable is measured repeatedly at different preset times for the same group of subjects or when subjects are exposed to all levels of the independent variable(s). The levels of an independent variable are called *within-subjects factors* and the design is called within-groups repeated measures ANOVA. For example, measuring the dependent variable at time 0, 5, 10, and 30 minutes after exposure to the independent variable. In this situation, time is the repeated factor with four levels, or measuring the subjects under levels of X, Y, and Z of the independent variable. The X, Y, and Z are called *within-subjects factors*.

In this design there is always one group of subjects who will be compared and will be undergoing different conditions of the independent variable. Usually the levels of independent variable are introduced to the subjects in a counterbalanced manner to rule out the order effect (learning, fatigue, or other changes due to previous exposure). Each subject acts as his or her own control and is compared for their response under different conditions (groups). Because the groups are the same, within group differences are no longer an issue in calculating the F ratio and the *Repeated Measure ANOVA*, which evaluates the differences between each group. This then requires different statistical analysis and computation of error. Most statistical packages such as SAS and SPSS do this analysis.

Multiple Comparison Tests

Analysis of variance and the *F* test show that there is a difference some place between the groups; however, it does not identify which group means are different from which. When an analysis of variance results in a significant *F*-ratio, the researcher must then carry out a multiple comparison test to find out which mean is significantly different from the other means. The type of test to be used may be decided before the ANOVA (priori) or after the analysis is done (post-hoc). Therefore, there are two types of multiple comparison tests.

a. Post hoc, or Posteriori, Multiple Comparison Tests

b. Priori, or Planned comparisons, Multiple Comparison Tests

a. Post Hoc or Posteriori. These tests are performed after analysis of variance has been completed. These are considered unplanned comparisons.

Types

➤ Tukey's honestly significant difference test
➤ Newman-Keuls test
➤ Duncan's new multiple range test
➤ Scheffe's Comparison
➤ Fisher's Least Significant Difference

b. Priori or Planned Comparisons. These tests are planned prior to data collection and will be performed even if the F-test is not significant based on the research rational.

Types
➤ Bonferroni-t-test
➤ Orthogonal contrasts
➤ Dunnet's test

Each multiple comparison test has its own characteristics and it is up to the researcher to decide which test to use. Most statistical analysis packages will perform the multiple comparison tests for you if it is found that the ANOVA is significant.

NON-PARAMETRIC TESTS

Non-parametric tests are used with lower levels of measurement such as nominal or ordinal data and are involved more with ranking than with comparisons. Overall, they are less sensitive. Non-parametric statistics also test the hypotheses for group comparisons without the assumptions for normality or variance. The outcomes of these tests are also evaluated according to predetermined alpha levels of significance.

Types:
A. Tests used with 2 correlated samples:
      -- Wilcoxon signed-rank test
      -- Sign test
B. Tests used with more than 2 correlated samples:
      -- Kruksal Wallis one-way analysis of variance
      -- Mann-Whitney U test
      -- Friedman two-way analysis of variance by rank

These tests are comparable to the t-test and ANOVA for parametric tests. Most statistical packages have these computations and are done easily.

ANALYSIS OF FREQUENCIES: CHI- SQUARE (X^2)

Chi-square (pronounced kye-square) is a commonly used non-parametric test and is mostly used for analyzing nominal data for frequency counts. This analysis is a comparison between expected frequencies (predicted scores based on the null hypothesis, or theoretical probability), and observed frequencies (what is actually occurring, or empirical probability).

Empirical probability. Is derived from the observation of certain events. By counting the frequency of occurrences, future projections could be made. All of the different chi-square statistical tests involve arranging the frequency distribution of the data in a contingency table of rows and columns. Estimates of error in predicting unit pairs in the rows and columns (based on the null hypothesis) are computed, subtracted from one another, and expressed in the form of a ratio or contingency coefficient.
The X^2 is a test to see if there is a significant deviation from what is expected to occur and what is actually happening.

$$X^2 = \frac{\sum(O\text{-}E)^2}{E}$$

O= observed frequency
E= expected frequency

Chi-square tests can easily be done by hand, or run using a statistical analysis package on a computer. The chi-square test for contingency is interpreted as the strength of the association measured, while the chi-square test for independence (which requires two samples) is a non-parametric test of significance to rule out sampling error and chance as much as possible.

Example: What is the expected number of males and females who enter the town library in one day? You would expect that the same number of males and females should be using the library (E = expected frequency, 50% male and 50% female), however your data may indicate otherwise (O = observed frequency). You would use the Chi-Square to see if there is a difference between your expected outcome and your observed outcome.

# of men entering the town library in one day = 56
# of women entering the library in one day = 44
Expected frequency: 50/50.

Gender	O	E	O-E	(O-E) 2	(O-E)2/E
Male	56	50	6	36	.55
Female	44	50	-6	36	.55
	100	100			

$X^2=\sum (O\text{-}E)^2/E=1.10$

When referring to critical values for chi-square at $\alpha = .05$ and one degree of freedom, the reported table value (0.05) X^2 (1_{df}) $=3.84$ is higher than the computational value and the null hypothesis is not rejected.

Table values could be found in most statistical analysis books or may be computed by computer statistical packages.

SUMMARY

Statistics play a significant role in making sense out of the data you collect. Probabilities estimate whether or not your differences are "true" or due to chance. Statistics provide you with the tools to determine if your hypothesis can be supported. The power of a statistical test is determined by several factors and needs to be decided upon prior to data collection. Depending on the levels of measurement and statistical assumption, you should choose the right statistical analysis approach for your data. Statistical packages, such as SAS and SPSS, will perform all the analyses for you as long as you provide the correct information.

EXERCISES

1. Create 3 non-directional hypotheses that relate to a health issue/topic of your interest (make sure they make sense!).
2. Create 3 directional hypotheses that relate to a health issue/topic of your interest (make sure they make sense!).
3. What is the difference between parametric and non-parametric statistics?
4. What does α, β, $1-\alpha$, and $1-\beta$ mean and how are they related to the power of a statistical test?
5. The power of a statistical test is the function of what four criterions?
6. What is the difference between the F ratio and the t ratio?
7. When do you use multiple comparison tests?
8. What is the difference between correlation and regression?
9. In Chi-Square, X^2, what does Empirical Probability mean?

QUESTIONS FOR DISCUSSION

1. A researcher randomly assigns her subjects to three groups for her experimental study. The dependant variable that she is measuring is the subjects' blood pressure. What types of statistical analyses are most appropriate for this study? She is thinking about multiple t-tests. Is this a good idea? Why or why not?

2. A Pearson-Moment-Correlation Coefficient analysis found that r was significant at 0.4. Should the researcher take this result and present it as a strong relationship? What else can he do to look at the relationships between his two variables?

FOR STUDENTS DOING THEIR RESEARCH

1- What types of statistical tests will you be doing for your data analysis? Are they going to be parametric or non-parametric? Why?

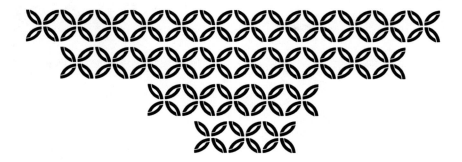

NOTES

PART VI

RESEARCH ETHICS
&
COMMUNICATION

CHAPTER (17)   Ethical Issues in Research
CHAPTER (18)   Research Proposal Writing
CHAPTER (16)   Research Communication

CHAPTER

17

ETHICAL ISSUES IN RESEARCH

OVERALL OBJECTIVE

To develop an understanding of the role of ethics in conducting research

GOALS

1. Define ethics and major issues in ethical research
2. Describe sources of misconduct/issues in ethical research
3. Describe the responsibilities of an ethical researcher
4. Comprehend the historical basis for ethical conduct
5. Describe sources for our code of ethics
6. Identify review process procedures and elements of the informed consent form

DEFINITION OF ETHICS

The word ethics is derived from the Greek word "ethos" meaning character, custom or usage, or morality and from the Latin synonym, meaning manner, custom, or habit. Ethics is the study of normative behavior. It is what we should and ought to do and what is right and wrong when involving in our conducts. The purpose of research ethics is to identify problems that arise while conducting research. The conduct of research gives rise to countless ethical questions. These questions arise from the study question, design, data collection, and reporting of findings. The goal of research ethics is to 1) determine the appropriateness of specific conduct and 2) establish actions and moral norms that a moral agent ought to take in a particular situation.

Considerations of Ethical Issues in Research

Every investigator has a moral responsibility for honesty and veracity during all stages of the research process. Some issues such, as deception, intent to defraud, and dishonesty are sometimes relatively straightforward. However, some issues are harder and less straightforward, for example:

➢ What types of data should be included when reporting the research?
➢ Who should be included as an author?
➢ When is a researcher should be allowed to use deception as part of the research procedures?
➢ What data should be considered as outliers?

The number of instances of research misconduct is higher than the number reported. This is due to researchers not knowing what should be reported. Whether it is their responsibility to report somebody else's conduct, and to whom they should report without jeopardizing their own situations. For these reasons, the Federal government now has specific measures for handling allegations of research misconduct and encourages reporting of misconduct by those who observe it. Most recently, the NIH, the NSF, and other funding agencies encourage education in the responsibility of ethical research conduct for all researchers.

[It is recommended that students take the online course on ethical issues on human subjects' research from the NIH website. The NIH website is: http://cme.nci.nih.gov/. Go to the site and follow the directions.]

Major Issues in Unethical Research

1. Ignorance
2. Stress
3. Research Misconduct
4. Witnessing Misconduct

1. **Ignorance.** Some unethical conduct stems from simple ignorance. For example:

➢ Not understanding how to cite resources properly in a report
➢ Not knowing if an idea is common or must be attributed
➢ Not knowing how to define an outlier in research
➢ Not knowing the policies and procedures regarding research conduct on human or animal subjects

Researchers have an ethical responsibility to conduct unbiased research and must report their results completely and with honestly. Resources used must be cited correctly and if there is doubt whether an idea is common knowledge or should be cited, it is better to acknowledge the idea with a proper citation. Researchers also have the responsibility to learn all policies and procedures involving the conduct of research in their institutions, especially those policies regarding human subjects and animal research.

2. Stress. One of the major sources of unethical conduct in research is stress. Due to a significant amount of pressure imposed on researchers especially at universities, with the motto of *"Publish or Perish!"* just doing something can seem more important than how it is done. This may put stress on an individual to do something unethical. Sometimes the excitement of reporting the results and rushing through the research process may give rise to the potential for unethical conduct. For example, what if you are "certain" that you have the right conclusion now and it can potentially save lives, even though you have not collected all the pertinent data?

Sometimes a researcher may want to publish his or her results in a journal publication. However, page limits imposed by these journals make it difficult for the researcher to "tell everything". This may force the researcher to only report positive or supportive results and not talk about the data that was not supportive of the research hypothesis. On the other hand, slicing up the results of a study to produce multiple papers may give rise to unethical conduct by trying to increase the number of publications.

ADVICE:
"BE PATIENT". Reporting wrong data or inaccuracy in reporting the research will eventually catch up with you in later life.

3. Research Misconduct. The three major issues in research misconduct are:

1. *Fabrication:* Producing non-existing data
2. *Falsification:* Changing the existing data to support the research hypothesis or to misguide the funding agency
3. *Plagiarism:* Copying material from others and reporting it as your own

These are clear-cut wrong practices. Any person who gets involved in these activities will seriously damage their research career and life. Even if the conduct seems minor at the time, it could penalize the person harshly later in life.

4. Witnessing Research Misconduct: *If you witness unethical behavior in others what should you do?*

A clear difference between unethical behavior and an honest error is not always obvious. Overall, people make mistakes and not all mistakes are an indication of unethical behavior. Therefore, when you witness misconduct, first you must make sure that what you see is correct. It is better to give the person who appears to be involved in misconduct the benefit of the doubt first, it is possible that what you think is happening might not be what is actually happening. It is also important to understand, that your approach might be different, depending on whom you witnessed doing the misconduct: Is he or she a student, a colleague, or a mentor? It is better to approach the person and ask for an explanation without accusing the person than being confrontational. The most important thing is that no matter who is doing the misconduct, if you are sure, it is your ethical responsibility to report it.

GOOD VS. ETHICAL RESEARCH

There is no distinctive line between doing good research and doing ethical research. Sound research is concerned with the truthfulness and dependability of design and data. Ethical research is concerned with the data collection procedures, the social, physical, psychological, economical aspects of the discovery, issues related to harm to human or animal subjects, and attention to the welfare of others.

ETHICAL RESPONSIBILITY OF THE RESEARCHER

There are six major responsibilities that all researchers should be aware of while conducting research and these are:

  A. Scientific contribution of research
  B. Personal bias in measurement
  C. Publication of findings/manipulations
  D. Conflict of interest
  E. Authorship's acknowledgment
  F. Control group

A. *Scientific Contribution of Research.* Clinical research must be initiated and completed with the main idea that they are supposed to make significant contributions to the overall health of society. Research that does not make any scientific contribution should be avoided. The potential benefits and risks must be considered and the benefits must always prevail over the risks. All research must be done with a proposed sound design and observation of variables that are relevant to the question being asked. Finally, a competent person must always perform the research.

B. *Personal bias in Measurement.* Researchers must assure that personal bias is not affecting the results. Both unconscious and conscious biases may influence the reporting of data. This may support or not support the research hypothesis. Researchers must be aware of these issues and develop appropriate research protocols and design strategies to control for the bias in the research. Interactions between the researcher and the subjects should also be minimized, if such interactions, alter the subject's response to treatment. Although, we may not be able to completely eliminate the bias from research, we have to control it as much as possible.

C. *Publication of findings/manipulation.* Researchers have an obligation to publish the results of their research honestly, truthfully, and in detail. Statistical procedures used to manipulate data should be appropriate and should be used exclusively to obtain scientific results. All data should be included in the analysis, and only true differences should be reported.

D. *Conflict of Interest.* Researchers should be aware of potential conflicts of interest and know who will control the data collected during the research. It should be clear as to who owns the data and who has access to it when the project is completed. In principle, the research data belongs to the agency that provides funding. Researchers should avoid research that has major conflicts of interest with the funding agency, especially private funding agencies. These conflicts may not allow the researcher to report honest and complete results of the study.

E. *Authorship's acknowledgment.* When reporting the results of a research project as a publication, those who are listed as authors on the paper should have major contributions to the project. Sometimes, lab directors may want their names in a paper even if they had a minimal impact. Those who helped with the project, but do not deserve the authorship should be acknowledged at the end of the paper. The order in which authors are listed in the byline should be discussed and agreed upon at the start of the project. It is customary that, the names appear on the byline of a research report according to the author's contribution to the project.

F. *Control Group.* For an experimental comparison, there is a need for a control group or placebo group. To determine if an intervention is responsible for change in behavior, one group would receive treatment, and another group will receive no treatment or a sham. By comparing outcomes, the researcher could decide if the intervention caused a significant change. If at the completion of the study, the intervention was effective, the researcher is ethically responsible to offer the treatment to the control group if he/she thinks that they may benefit from it.

PROTECTING HUMAN RIGHTS IN CLINICAL RESEARCH

When human subjects are used in clinical research, great care must be exercised to ensure that the rights of those human subjects are protected.

HISTORICAL BACKGROUND

The protection of human subjects in research and the guidelines for human experimentation evolved following some clear abuses in the past. During World War II, the Nazi's performed medical experiments between 1930-1940 in which prisoners in concentration camps were used as subjects, leading to the death or permanent damage of many. In the United States, many studies have been identified over the years that show clear abuse of human subjects in experimental research. The most infamous was the Tuskegee Syphilis Study, which was conducted from 1932-1972. This study, which was supported by the US Department of Health and Human Services, involved many African American men diagnosed with syphilis who did not receive proper treatment even after Penicillin was discovered and recognized as the medicine of choice to treat syphilis. In 1963, in Brooklyn, New York in the Jewish Chronic Hospital, elderly women were injected with cancer cells without their knowledge, for a study to develop a vaccine for cancer. These terrible clinical abuses of human subjects in research led to the development of the Code of Ethics that are now used to guide research involving human subjects.

CODE OF ETHICS

The first code of ethics was the *Nuremberg Code of 1947*, which evolved following the Nazi medical experimentations. The major point of this code was that human subjects must voluntarily consent to participate in a research study. Subjects must be fully informed on the procedures of the study, risks, and benefits involved with the study before consenting to participate. The Nuremberg Code also noted the importance of the competency of the investigator to perform a study.

The *Declaration of Helsinki* was adopted by the World Medical Association (WMA) in 1964 and was revised in 1975. The basic principles of this code state that there should be a review panel for any research study involving human subjects. The members of the review panel must not be associated with the proposed project and must independently review the research proposals.
Reports of research that have not been conducted according to the stated principles should not be accepted for publication. Researchers must clearly address how they acquired the informed consent; otherwise their papers should not be published. Issues, such as competency of the investigators, importance of the research, and acquiring the consent form before subject participation were other components of the Helsinki Declaration.

The last and the most comprehensive code of ethics for the protection of human subjects was the *Belmont Report*. The National Commission for the Protection of Human Subjects of Biomedical and Behavioral Research, established by the National Research Act, issued a report in 1978 that served as the basis for regulations affecting research sponsored by the federal government. The latest revision was carried out in October of 2000. Modeled guidelines, developed by specific disciplines and different professions, developed their own professional codes of ethics based on the Belmont Report.

The Belmont Report articulated three primary ethical principles upon which standards of ethical conduct in research are based:

1. Beneficence
2. Respect

3. Justice

According to the Belmont Report, commitment to the protection of human rights and dignity must be inherent in the design of any clinical research project.

1. **The Issue of Beneficence.** The issue of beneficence incorporates two important aspects of research involving human subjects:
Freedom from Harm (Hippocratic Oath of Medicine: "Do no harm."). The decision of human subjects as to whether to participate or not in a research project should be respected and efforts must be taken to protect their well being during a study. There should never be exploitation of subjects in research and subjects must be informed of all aspects of the research.

Liability for Negligence. The researcher is obligated to maximize the benefits and minimize the possible harms to the subjects. In situations when there is a possibility of harm to a subject, the researcher must justify the importance of the benefits despite the possibility of harm and risk. Harmonizing the risks and benefits is a very important concern in research. However, a researcher should never withhold a medically necessary treatment.

2. **Principle of Respect.** The principle of respect for people incorporates the following ethical convictions:

Self-Determination: Individuals should be treated as autonomous agents.
Autonomy: "An autonomous person is an individual capable of deliberation about personal goals and of acting under such deliberation. To respect autonomy is to give weight to the autonomous persons' considered opinions and choices while refraining from obstructing their actions..." (The Belmont Report).

Research subjects must voluntarily participate in a research study after they are provided detailed information regarding the study and their involvement in the study. They should not be coerced into participating in a study and must be given enough time to make their decision. Special provisions must be made for persons with diminished autonomy and level of comprehension such as children, and people with severe developmental disorders and dementias. Researchers must give these people the opportunity to make their own decisions and, in cases of severe comprehension problems, the subjects' permission may be requested from other parties such as a child's parents, or legal guardians.

3. **Principle of Justice.** The ethical principle for justice requires that subjects have the right to fair treatment. The investigator must balance the risks and benefits ratio and the benefits of a study must overcome the risks. Researchers should not involve subjects in a research study if the subjects do not benefit from it unless there is clear justification for doing such a study. When doing a research study, the researcher must give an equal opportunity for participation in the study to all classes of subjects, regardless of gender, race, and age unless there is a clear justification for the inclusion or exclusion of a particular group of subjects.

The issue of justice also points to the importance of protecting the subjects' right to privacy and confidentiality of the information obtained from the subjects during the research study. Researchers must explain in detailed procedures that they will follow to protect subjects' confidentiality and anonymity.

Standardization of Ethical Principals

In response to the historical revelations after projects such as the Tuskegee study, the Department of Health and Human Services (DHHS) appointed a panel to review the Tuskegee study as well as the Department's policies and procedures for the protection of human participants in general. The panel proposed that Congress establish "a permanent board with the authority to regulate at least all federally supported research involving human subjects." As a result, the National Research Act was passed in 1974. This Act required the establishment of The National Commission for the Protection of Human *Institutional Review Boards (IRB)* to review all DHHS funded research. Subjects of Biomedical and Behavioral Research was also created by this Act. This Commission issued the Belmont Report, which provides ethical principles for biomedical and clinical research that must be followed by all institutions doing research involving human subjects. As a result, procedures to ensure the protection of human subjects in research have been delineated and are considered "standard" throughout the United States. Based on these principles, every study must have a research proposal. The research proposal must identify...

1. The problem or question to be studied
2. The rationale, need for, and importance of the study
3. Designs that are clearly stated and appropriate to answer the research question
4. Explanation as to why human subjects are needed for the study
5. How informed consent will be obtained

Institutional Review Board (IRB)

Each institution that is involved with clinical or biomedical research involving human subjects must have an IRB Committee. Members of the IRB should be men and women with adequate knowledge of research practices with no vested interest in the research study or its outcomes. Their responsibility is to assure that all research studies are ethical and justified. Each IRB must have at least five members with different backgrounds and should include people of different gender, ethnicity, race, as well as those sensitive to community attitudes. Each IRB should include at least one member whose primary concern is in a scientific area and one member whose primary concern is in a nonscientific area. The IRB may have as many members as needed to perform a complete and adequate review of all research activities. As necessary, the IRB should consult with knowledgeable people regarding different issues that arise, including, but not limited to: children, prisoners, pregnant women, and disabled or cognitively impaired persons. These individuals are not voting members. Members should not be involved in reviewing research projects in which they have a conflict of interest.

Roles and Responsibilities of the IRB

An IRB protects the rights, safety, and welfare of human research participants by:

a) Reviewing all research protocols to ensure that they meet the criteria for the protection of human subjects.
b) Ratifying that the research plan does not expose subjects to unreasonable risks.
c) Ensuring that the purposes of the research and the setting in which the research will be conducted are mindful of the special problems of research involving vulnerable populations. Participants should equally share the foreseeable benefits and risks.
d) Ensuring that procedures for acquiring informed consent is appropriate and that the informed consent is sought from each prospective participant or the participant's legally authorized representative.
e) Seeing that the researcher provides adequate provisions to protect the privacy of the participants and maintains the confidentiality of data.

In situations where the participants are likely to be vulnerable to coercion or undue influence (e.g., children, prisoners, pregnant women, mentally disabled, economically or educationally disadvantaged persons), the researcher must adequately explain what additional safeguards are included in the study to protect the rights and welfare of these participants.

Assessment of Risks and Benefits

Risks to subjects are classified as physical, psychological, social, and economical. The risks may be considered minimal or more than minimal risks. Minimal risk is when the magnitude of harm or discomfort from the research is not greater than those ordinarily encountered in daily life or during the performance of routine physical or psychological examinations or tests. The concept of minimal risk is used by the IRB to decide whether the project should have a full review or not. The benefit from research is classified as new knowledge to improve the health of the participants and for the general population.

Types of IRB Review

Depending on the level of risk involved with the research protocol, the IRB can ask for a full board review, expedited review, or exempt from review.

Expedited review: For research that involves no more than minimal risk and for minor changes in previously approved research, the IRB chair or a designated voting member, or group of voting members, review the proposed research rather than the full IRB. If a research involves a survey or interview with sensitive questions that may cause psychological harm or distress in subjects, it will be considered more than minimal risk and should not be processed under expedited review.

Full Review: For research that is considered to have more than minimal risk, there should be a full board review. For this process, the researcher must submit a proposal to the IRB. The research proposal is presented and discussed at a full IRB meeting when a quorum of members is present. For the research to be approved, it must receive the approval of a majority of the voting members present.

Exempt from IRB Review: Certain low-risk research is exempt from the IRB review. The following are the six exempt categories as listed in 45CFR46.101(b) of the Federal Regulations:

1. Research conducted in established or commonly accepted educational settings, involving normal educational practices.
2. Research involving the use of educational tests (cognitive, diagnostic, aptitude, achievement), survey procedures, interview procedures, or observation of public behavior, unless:
   a. Information obtained is recorded in such a manner that human participants can be identified, directly or through identifiers linked to the participants; and/or
   b. Any disclosure of the human participant's responses outside the research could reasonably place the participants at risk of criminal or civil liability or be damaging to the participant's financial standing, employability or reputation.
3. Research involving the use of educational tests (cognitive, diagnostic, aptitude, achievement), survey procedures, interview procedures, or observation of public behavior that is not exempt under paragraph (2) of this section, if:
   a. The participants are elected or appointed public officials or candidates for public office; or
   b. Federal statute(s) require(s) without exception that the confidentiality of the personally identifiable information will be maintained throughout the research and thereafter.
4. Research involving the collection or study of existing data, documents, records, pathological specimens or diagnostic specimens, if these sources are publicly available or if the information is recorded by the researcher in such a manner that participants cannot be identified, directly or through identifiers linked to the participants.
5. Research and demonstration projects which are conducted by or subject to the approval of Department or Agency heads, and which are designed to study, evaluate, or otherwise examine public health benefit or service programs.
6. Taste and food quality evaluation and consumer acceptance studies.

These exemptions do not apply to research involving prisoners, fetuses, pregnant women or human in vitro fertilization. Further, the exemption in item two (above), does not apply to children, except for research involving observations of public behavior when the researcher(s) do not participate in the activities being observed.

The IRB has the authority to:

1. Approve, disapprove, or terminate all research activities that fall within its jurisdiction according to relevant federal regulations and local institutional policy;
2. Require modifications in protocols, including previously approved research;
3. Require additional information be provided to the research participants when the IRB deems that this information would add to the protection of their rights and welfare;
4. Require documentation of informed consent or allow waiver of documentation, in accordance with article 45CFR46.117.

Elements of Informed Consent

The informed consent form must be written in a lay language that can be understood by a person with a second grade education. It should include the following:

1. Title of the Study
2. Name of the Investigators and their Affiliations
3. Purpose of the Study: Must be clearly stated, so subjects understand why their participation in the study is needed.
4. Process of Data Collection: Process of data collection should be explained to the subjects and, if possible, complex medical words should be avoided or explained in a lay language. The subject should know how long they will be involved in the study and what procedures they are expected to go through.
5. Inclusion/Exclusion Criteria: Inclusion and exclusion criteria for selecting the subjects should be explained so participants understand why they have been chosen to participate in the research.
6. Risks/Benefits: All risks including (physical, social, psychological, and economical) should be explained. The researcher must explain how they plan to minimize the risks and what types of safeguards they are offering to protect the subjects. Possible benefits from the research to the study participants or general population should also be explained.
7. Alternative Treatment: Subjects must be informed of all the possible alternative treatments available to them. They should have the freedom to decide if they want to receive the alternative treatments.
8. Confidentiality/Anonymity: The researcher should explain how the anonymity and confidentiality of the subjects would be protected. Sentences such as "the subjects will be given random numbers", or "the data will only be available to the principle investigators" should be included. Subjects must be assured that their names or personal information will not be disclosed in any publication arising from the research.

9. Freedom to Withdraw: The consent form should have a section indicating that subjects voluntarily participate in the study and that they have the right to withdraw from the study at any time, without the fear of prejudice or unfair treatment by the investigators.

10. Children & Minors/Prisoners/Pregnant Women: If research involves any of these vulnerable populations, care must be taken to assure their autonomy and the researcher must explain how they plan to protect these subjects. Children in research are individuals up to age of 18 years. Any time a child is involved in research, either a parent, if available, or a legal guardian must sign the consent form. Any child 7 years and older must also sign a consent form individually.

ETHICAL ISSUES IN ANIMALS RESEARCH

The major advancements in medical and biomedical research during the last few years have been through the use of animal studies. While scientists recognize the need for animals as study subjects, they also express concerns about the humane use of animals for research. A major concern has always been needless suffering, humane or non-humane.

There are criteria that should always guide investigators in assessing the use of animal subjects for a research study. Before a researcher starts a study involving animal subjects, he or she must answer the following questions:

1. Are animals necessary to perform this specific study?
2. Can the researcher identify similar studies on the same species of animal so that he or she can use the data collected on those studies rather than sacrificing a new group of animals?
3. How can the researcher assure that the animal species selected and the number of animals proposed to use in the study is appropriate?
4. Can computer modeling be used to do the study rather than live animals?
5. How important is the scientific contribution of this study to justify the money and number of animals that will be used to answer the question?

After justification and answering the above questions, the researcher must carefully plan and use animals in research. The researcher is responsible and accountable to propose a study that has quality and value. Attention must be paid to the selection of appropriate species, as well as careful determination of the number of animals needed for accurate data collection. The researcher must identify how proper care, including food, housing, and overall attention to well being, will be provided and whether he or she has the environment and resources to do so. All procedures must be performed to prevent animal suffering as much as possible. If necessary, anesthetics must be provided. If the animal should be sacrificed, careful consideration must be given regarding humane procedures to end life.

TYPES OF ANIMAL RESEARCH

Animal research can be performed either in-vitro or in-vivo. In-vitro research involves the use of isolated cells and organelles from the body and experimenting with those tissues outside of the body. For example, isolated intestinal segments. In-vivo research involves experimenting with animals by performing a procedure. For example, catheterized animal models, balance studies using animals, or isotopic food labeling.

Advantages: The advantage of using animals in research is that these experiments are:

1. Relatively easy to prepare and perform in various locations.
2. Animals multiply and grow fast; thus, the number of subjects and duration of the study are not problematic.
3. Many techniques that cannot be performed on humans due to health, safety, ethical, and cost considerations can be conducted using animal subjects.

Disadvantages: The disadvantages of animal research are:

1. Questionable applicability to humans (the results must be extrapolated with great care).
2. In situations when in-vitro research involves the use of body parts outside of the body where normal hormonal and perfusion are interrupted, the results should be observed with caution.
3. Experiments on anesthetized animals do not simulate normal physiological conditions.

Researchers must follow the following 3 principals when conducting animal research (referred to as the program of "3Rs"):

A. Reduction--- The number of animals used in research should be reduced. Some of the procedures that a researcher can use to reduce the number of animals as much as possible are:

➤ Literature review (review the previous research related to the investigation and the number of animals used in those studies. If possible use the data from those studies).
➤ Use statistical significance and power analysis to estimate the number of animals needed to reach desired levels of significance.
➤ Use disease free animals (this will reduce attrition and help with maintaining the sample size for statistical significance).
➤ Share animals or tissues with other researchers (this will prevent others from sacrificing more animals).

B. Refinement---These are techniques used to reduce stress and pain in animals. Use protocols that ensure that death is not the end point; reduce pain, by using anesthesia, analgesics, or tranquilizers. Animals should be cared for after surgical procedures including keeping them warm, providing antibiotics and analgesics as needed, and removing the sutures in a timely fashion.

C. Replacement--- These are techniques that replace the use of animals for research. For example, using animal models or computer simulations for research. Before experimenting with live animals, practice new techniques on cadavers first.

INSTITUTIONAL ANIMAL CARE AND USE COMMITTEE (IACUC)

Each institution involved in animal research must have an IACUC. The committee should be composed of at least five members; one member should not be affiliated with the institution and another member must be a veterinarian. This committee evaluates research for the humane treatment of animals, study design, procedures to be used, and care of the animals. Any research involving animals must be approved by the IACUC before initiation.

Laboratory Inspections
Public Health Services Policy (PHS) and the Animal Welfare Regulations (AWR) require that the Institutional Animal Care and Use Committee (IACUC) inspect, at least once every six months, all animal facilities including animal study areas. All laboratories and areas where animals are brought for use in experiments must be inspected and approved by the IACUC. Routine IACUC inspections are unannounced as are visits by Federal officials. All laboratory or farm animals must be treated humanely, fed properly, and given adequate veterinary care.

Activities Exempt from Protocol for Animal Care
1. Use of dead animals or tissues
2. Non-invasive observations of wild animals in their natural habitat
3. Routine livestock procedures for the maintenance of the animals and are not part of an experiment per se (vaccinations, castration)

SUMMARY

Ethics define how we conduct our behavior and ethical research defines how we conduct research that is morally right. As a researcher, you should be aware of ethical issues in research and must pursue and understand your ethical responsibilities. Misconduct in research is a grave offense. History illustrates a basis for ethical requirements. The review processes for both human and animal research helps us to be aware of our ethical responsibilities.

EXERCISES

2- What is the relationship between academic freedom and research ethics? What are the considerations?

3- Find some additional historical ethical issues other than what was discussed in this chapter.

4- What is the difference between anonymity and confidentiality?

5- What does IRB stand for?

6- A research study involves evaluating the reading ability of a group of second grade school children in their classroom. Do you need to have a consent form? Why? Why not?

7- What is the program of the "3R's"?

8- Is it ethical to tell subjects that they are free to withdraw from the study at any time?

QUESTIONS FOR DISCUSSION

1- What do you regard as your primary defense against unethical conduct in research?

2- A researcher studies the sex lives of people who are HIV positive (with their consent). During the course of the study interviews, some subjects identify other individuals who have not provided informed consent. Does this raise ethical concerns? What, if anything, can the researcher do to protect the other individuals?

3- A professor asks her students to participate in her study but does not explain the study and the procedures. If you were one of those students, would you ask for more information before participating? Would you feel pressured to participate because you want to please your professor?

FOR STUDENTS WHO ARE PLANNING TO DO RESEARCH

1- Does your study involve the use of human subjects? If so, do you anticipate any harm to the participants? What measures will you take to protect the subjects in your study?

2- Does your study involve animal subjects? If so, how are you planning to follow the program of the 3R's?

NOTES

CHAPTER

18

RESEARCH PROPOSAL WRITING

OVERALL OBJECTIVES

To become familiar with research planning for the purpose of proposal writing and applying the skills learned to your own areas of experience and expertise.

GOALS

1. Describe the research proposal and identify its purposes
2. Delineate the components of a research plan
3. Become familiar with the steps in creating a research plan for the development of a research proposal
4. Discuss different components of the proposal and their significance

THE RESEARCH PROPOSAL

The research process begins with identifying a research question and defining the methods and procedures needed to collect appropriate data to answer the question with accuracy and confidence. The success of research depends on how well in advance these elements have been determined. The Research Proposal is a written plan that describes the process of identifying the research question, the rational for the study, and the methods and procedures to collect and analyze the data in order to find the answer to the question. The research proposal is an important part of any research process. No research should be carried out without first writing a well thought out research proposal.

A proposal is used to describe the...

➤ Purpose of the study
➤ The importance of the research question
➤ The research protocol
➤ Feasibility of the project

Every research proposal has two basic parts: 1) *the research plan* and 2) *the administrative plan.* The research plan is a step-by-step description of the researcher's scientific approach to finding the answer to the research question. The administrative plan is the description of resources needed to perform the study (personnel, equipment, and environment) and how the researcher plans to manage the money that the funding agency will provide to him or her to do the study. In summary, a researcher must be a scientist (knows his or her area of research), a sales person (be able to sell his or her idea/s to a funding agency by providing the rational and proper methodology), and a good manger (be able to efficiently manage the grant money). All of these aspects must be explained in the research proposal.

PURPOSES OF A RESEARCH PROPOSAL

A research proposal is an indispensable part of any research and can serve many purposes during a study, including:

1. Representing the knowledge and understanding of the researcher with regards to the scientific area under investigation and the existing literature.
2. Indicating that the assumptions and rationale proposed by the researcher is correct.
3. Demonstrating that the methods chosen for the study are appropriate to answer the question.
4. Providing necessary information for a grant application.
5. Serving as an application for IRB review.
6. Enhancing communication between researchers involved with the study.
7. Serving as a guide for data collection.

STEPS IN DEVELOPING A RESEARCH PROPOSAL

Before you start to write a research proposal there are steps that should be followed.

Step 1: Initiating the idea
Initiating an idea, or finding a research problem, requires that you---
Become aware of research problems in your clinical field. Find ways to read and increase your understanding for research problems. Identify and define a question in the problem area that is answerable through appropriate research methodology.

Step 2: Selecting the problem

Finding the source of a research problem varies according to your personal experiences. In general the process begins with an idea or a need. The idea or need is then translated to a specific problem to be studied.

Beginning researchers often confuse **a problem** with a **problem area.**

Problem areas are vague as to a specific problem. Each problem area contains innumerable research problems. For example, if you are a dietitian and would like to do research on obesity, obesity is a problem area that in itself is vague. You should specify one problem in this area and focus your research on that specific problem. For example, you may want to study the relationship between high blood pressure and obesity in older adults. This is now a problem.

To find a research problem: 1) read studies in your field, 2) analyze statements made in professional journals, 3) analyze and review those studies that you are not satisfied with, 4) browse the reference lists in books, journals, magazines, and theses. Sometimes just reading the title of studies in the reference section of an article may spark a viable idea for research. After you identify your problem, you should proceed with step 3.

Step 3: Initial review of literature

You should start to read as many research articles as possible related to your problem or research question. The purpose of this review of literature is to develop an understanding of the current body of knowledge concerning your problem. This is the specific, extensive, and systematic examination of resources to help you understand and discover what has been studied, what is known and what needs to be investigated.

This initial review of literature will allow you to examine different methodologies that were used by others, including processes of subject selection, sample size determination, types of instruments that have been used to collect similar data, and data analysis techniques. It will help you to identify your variables and how to define them. Based on the experiences of other researchers, you may be able to determine the potential for a successful outcome of your study and estimate the likelihood that your planned project will accomplish its objectives.

Sources for a Review of Literature

1. Bibliography
2. Abstracts
3. Indexes
4. Research reviews
5. Journals
6. Computerized information retrieval

In summary, the literature review should be done *continuously* throughout the project. However, the majority should be performed *before the final plan* for conducting the research project.

Step 4: Defining the problem

Following the initial review of literature, develop a specific statement of the problem, why the problem is important and how the problem is delimited.

Once you have an idea for a problem, consult the literature again to obtain additional background information that will help you to define the problem more specifically. This is especially true in regard to obtaining ideas about methods, techniques, and instrumentation needed to attack the problem.

Before you invest time and resources to start a research project on a specific problem, ask the following questions:

1. Is this a unique problem?
2. Is it worth your time and money to study this problem?
3. Will it add to the existing knowledge base?
4. Is it substantial?
5. Is it feasible/practical?
6. Is it ethical?
7. Is it timely?
8. Are you sufficiently trained to conduct the study?

If the answers to the above questions are positive, select a research approach and determine whether the problem will be attacked descriptively, correlationally, or experimentally. Determining your methods and techniques will supply the needed research data. During this process consider cost, demands made on the research subjects, and the level of skill possessed by the researcher.

Step 5: State the hypothesis

Determine the expected outcome of your study based upon the literature and your experience by proposing appropriate hypothesis (es). Hypotheses are tentative conclusions, intelligent/educated guesses before all the facts are established, especially in experimental and correlational research. The purpose of experimental and correlational research is to test hypotheses and, ultimately, provide evidence so that the researcher can accept or reject the hypotheses.

Characteristics of a Hypothesis

1. Declarative statement that predicts the relationship between the independent & dependent variables
2. Usually incorporates phrases such as "greater than", "less than", "different from" or "related to"
3. Must be able to observe & measure the dependent & independent variables
4. Must be acceptable and based on sound rationale
5. A body of knowledge should support the hypothesis

Step 6: Finalize your plan

At this time you should be able to answer the following questions:

1. Have you identified your population and sample for your study?
2. What types of subjects will produce the needed research data?
3. Are the subjects appropriate?
4. How many subjects are needed?
5. How will they be selected?
6. What instrumentation do your methods and techniques require?
7. What are the costs and demands on the subjects?
8. What is the availability and adequacy of your instruments?
9. Have you developed the data-collecting plan, data-analysis plan, and identified the statistical procedures needed?
10. Do you have enough knowledge and professional expertise to do this research?

Suggested Actions...

Conduct pilot studies of the approach, methods, instruments, and data-analysis plan. Perform a trial run of the procedures to be sure that everything works. If problems develop, revise the procedures as needed.

Step 7: Determining potential for successful outcomes
Based on previous work by others and your pilot testing, estimate the likelihood that your project will accomplish its objectives. If previous research has failed, ask different questions or look at different measuring tools.

COMPONENTS OF THE RESEARCH PROPOSAL

Each funding agency may require different headings or sub-headings for a grant proposal depending on their format. However, in general, most research proposals follow the following format with some minor differences.

A. PROPOSAL IDENTIFICATION SECTION

1. Title of the Research Study
2. Name and Title of Investigator(s) & Participating Facilities

B. RESEARCH PLAN SECTION

1. Abstract
2. Introduction
3. Objectives/Specific Aims
4. Hypotheses
5. Review of Literature
6. Need/Significance of the Study/Application
7. Methodology
8. Limitations and Delimitations

9. Bibliography or References

C. ADMINISTRATIVE PLAN SECTION

1. Time, Space and Availability of Equipment
2. Budget
3. Informed Consent Procedures

A. PROPOSAL IDENTIFICATION SECTION

The Title:

The title of the study is the FIRST thing seen by readers and is often the last decision made by the researcher in planning the study. The title is the project's *"public identity"* and provides the first impression of what the reader should expect to read in the subsequent pages.

It has to be concise and informative. Most funding agencies limit the number of characters in the title (56-60 including the spaces). The title should be long enough to cover the subject of the research, but short enough to be interesting. When you select a title for your research project ask the following questions of your title...

➢ Is it precise enough to identify the problem?
➢ Is it clear, concise, and adequately descriptive to put the study in its proper category?
➢ Are the important key words properly used?
➢ Are unnecessary words eliminated to make it more interesting?
➢ Are the most important words at the beginning?

Example: "Isometric exercise and bone mass in post menopausal women"
This title has 51 characters (62 with spaces), the independent variable is Isometric exercises, the dependent variable is bone mass and the population under study is postmenopausal women. This is a very concise and informative title.

B. RESEARCH PLAN SECTION

1- The Abstract

The abstract is a summary of the research project and is usually limited to one page (150-200 words). The funding agencies and institutional review boards always require an abstract or summary. Sometimes some funding agencies require the abstract in a lay language, so that it is understandable by all (not just the scientific community) who are affected by this type of research. The abstract is also the public identity of a research project and some reviewers first read the abstract to see whether the project merits a full review or not. Therefore, an abstract must convey specifically what is to be done and the importance of the problem.

In general an abstract should highlight:

➤ The purpose and importance of the proposed project
➤ A brief description of the project methodology (subjects, procedures, methods, and data analysis) and proposed duration
➤ Cost and specific objectives of the project

2- Introduction/Rationale

The introduction of the proposal is a brief one to two paragraphs describing the problem. It is more preferable that the content be based on the writer's own words and should make a positive impression on the reader. A good introduction should include the rationale conveying the importance of the problem (some references to the literature can be made). The statement of the problem comes immediately after the rationale and is a declarative statement indicating the research question. An introduction should be clear, concise, and definitive and include all of the problem elements and variables to be studied in terms of their relationship.

3- Purpose of the Study

The purpose of the study is one sentence indicating precisely what the project is expected to accomplish. It follows the justification presented in the introduction and the statement of the problem.

4- Objectives and Specific Aims

Objectives or specific aims (either term could be used) are outcomes that are measurable and should be achieved by the end of the study. Objectives can serve to: add to a body of knowledge in a certain content area, test a theoretical proposition, demonstrate differences between certain treatments, develop more effective and efficient intervention strategies, document the reliability of an instrument, establish the relationship between specific variables, and finally use the results in decision making for treatments.

5- Need for the Study

The need for the study or significance of the study, or justification of the study (terms used interchangeably depending on the format of the proposal), usually follows the objectives of the study, and is used to justify the study. Reviews of previous studies/literature may be used to justify the present research and to indicate why the study is needed. This section explains why the study is significant and tries to justify its contents.

Overall, this section will attempt to show that one or more of the following is true:

➤ There is a need to find an answer to this specific question
➤ There is a knowledge gap in this specific area

> ➤ More understanding of the phenomenon is needed
> ➤ The information available should be validated
> ➤ Clarifications are needed in regards to the current practices concerning the problem

6- Background/Review of Literature

The Background/Review of literature (either term may be used) section includes information about the theoretical rationale for the study. Pertinent facts, observations, or claims that have led the investigator to the proposed research question will be discussed with proper citation to the studies reviewed. The information in this section is derived mainly from the literature reviewed and from previous or related work done by the investigator (pilot testing). Funding agencies look favorably on projects that are built on previous work by the investigator.

Types of Literature Review

Primary References. These references are original articles, reports, or books written by experts or authorities in a problem area. They may offer ideas, operational definitions, and theories about what is good, bad, desirable or undesirable in the problem area. The researcher directly obtains these originals and reads them.

Secondary References. These references are those in which the original work is described/mentioned by someone other than the author of the original work (i.e., second hand information). For example, work may be mentioned in an original article by the author, and the researcher takes the author's word for that and uses that as a reference. Secondary referencing is not recommended during literature review. The researcher must make efforts to obtain the original work read and use them as references. However, in situations when the original work is not available (in microchips in another country), the use of these types of references might be justified.

Some practical recommendations for writing the review of literature section of your proposal:

When writing the review of literature, try to make a case for the importance of the proposed project and justify the need for the study based on what has been expressed by others. Present the material concisely and integrate published material to make relevant points in order to convince the reader of your grasp of the subject matter, address theory that supports the question, choice of variables, and how the outcome will be interpreted. You should never create a list of abstracts of all the articles you've read without your intellectual interpretation and how they support your proposal.

The literature review can be *frustrating* and not particularly an enjoyable activity! You have to spend a lot of time in the library. Conduct your review by looking at the most current literature first, and then work backwards. Familiarize yourself with newer methods, techniques, procedures, and instrumentation. Create a functional bibliography by listing the following information on index cards and note all bibliographic information for each source including:

> Author's last name and initials
> Title of the journal article, book, report or review
> Volume or issue number, year, month of the journal
> Publisher of the book, edition & date of publication
> Page number of the article or book referenced and the library call number

Make a working bibliography by:

> Identify each source in the working bibliography
> Evaluate the value of the source to your project
> References may be added or deleted depending on whether or not your research focus has changed
> Read valuable sources in depth
> Take notes during critical reading to ensure accuracy
> When sources disagree, both sides of the issue should be noted

During the write up of the review of literature do the followings:

> Thoroughly review the literature and organize notes for presentation in this part of the proposal
> Present an insightful analysis/evaluation of each research source as it relates to your objectives
> Justify your study, establish its worth and overall justification
> Don't include studies that do not have a significant relationship to the problem you are addressing
> Be *focused* and include related references to your research topic
> Site the current research, and whenever possible, include research done by reviewers of your proposal (if you know them)
> Propose what *research gap* you are planning to fill
> Critically evaluate existing knowledge, but do not fan the flames of scientific controversy. Nothing is to be gained from tearing apart someone else's research in your research proposal

7- Methodology

The methodology section of the proposal describes and justifies the design that the researcher proposes to use in order to answer the research question. It also describes the procedures to be utilized, including type of subjects and their selection process, testing protocols and instruments, data collection procedures, and data analysis procedures. This is considered the most important part of a proposal.

Components of the Methodology Section:

a) Design
b) Subject selection
c) Materials/Instruments
d) Development of the test instruments
e) Procedures for testing & gathering data
f) Statistical analysis

a) Design. A researcher could add to the body of knowledge utilizing several different types of designs. However, it is the research question that determines the research design. Usually, the general sequence of a research design if you know nothing or almost nothing about the topic, proceeds from:
> *Descriptive ---> Correlation ---> Predictive*

The sequence of a descriptive research design proceeds from:
> Qualitative (nominal) --->Normative form

The sequence of a predictive research design proceeds from:
> *Simple ---> Complex*

In the design section of the proposal, the researcher makes a case as to why he or she has chosen a specific design and why this is the best design to answer the research question accurately. The specifics of the design should be discussed (i.e., experimental, quasi experimental, qualitative descriptive, etc.).

b) Subject Selection. In this section, the researcher specifically describes the relevant characteristics of the subjects and how the characteristics of the subjects are appropriate for testing the proposed hypothesis. The process of recruiting subjects for the project (inclusion or exclusion of minorities and women in the study) as well as the inclusion and exclusion criteria for subject selection should be discussed. Sample size determination and power analysis, as well as plans to control for subject attrition, should also be discussed.

c) Materials/Instruments. Depending on the type of research the researcher may require different types of instruments to collect their data. The instrument could be something that is already available in the market and is a valid tool to measure the response variable. In these cases, the researcher should explain the instrument and provide information regarding the product (brand name, company's name and address). Sometimes the tool has to be developed by the researcher. For example, the researcher may be developing a survey or a questionnaire to measure some variable. In these cases, the researcher must explain thoroughly, why this is a valid tool to measure the response variable and how the validity and reliability of the tool was checked.

d) Procedures for testing and gathering data. The researcher should provide a detailed and chronological sequence of what is to be done from the beginning to the end of data collection procedures. Including, what, when, how, and by whom the data will be collected. This section should be written like a recipe book, meaning that all activities regarding data collection should be explained in detail, so that if someone unfamiliar with the project is going to duplicate the process he or she could do so without any difficulty. Usually the researcher creates a timetable of the procedural sequences. For example, if the researcher were proposing a three-year study, in the timetable he or she would explain what would happen during each week, month, quarter of the research process timeline.

e) Statistical Analyses/Data Collection. Based on the research design and the research question, the researcher should propose what type of statistical analysis will be performed to test the hypothesis (es). The data analysis should describe all of the procedures for collecting, recording, reducing, and analyzing the data. The researcher should also describe how the collected information becomes the data on which inferences will be drawn. Some points that should be discussed in this section depending on the design are:

➢ The level of measurement for each variable (nominal, ordinal, or metric)
➢ Justification for short and long-term data collection
➢ Justification for rater bias and subject/researcher interaction
➢ Consideration for respondent burden and steps to avoid collecting *side* data

Guiding Questions When Writing the Methodology

➢ Did you specify the population to be studied?
➢ Is the design appropriate to answer the research question?
➢ Was the sampling procedure and sample selection discussed? Is it appropriate for this study?
➢ How the control group was selected?
➢ How various treatments were assigned?
➢ Were appropriate statistical procedures and level of significance selected in advance?
➢ Can the design be replicated by others, is it clear?

8- Delimitation and Limitations

Sometimes a researcher includes a section in the research proposal to discuss the limitations and delimitations of the study. In the *delimitations*, the researcher talks about the scope of the study and draws a line around the study "fencing it in". He or she identifies what is included in the research and spells out what a researcher can control such as the number and kinds of subjects and variables, the tests/measures/instruments that will be used in the study, special equipment and/or type of training, time, duration of the study (# of weeks, dates), and analytical procedures. This is simply to communicate to the reader that, the researcher is aware of other approaches that could be used to do the research, but with the resources available this is the best approach to answer the question.

Limitations: In the limitations of the study, the researcher talks about the weaknesses of the study and matters that the researcher cannot control, but may influence the results of the study. Only issues that might affect the acceptability of the research data should be presented. Statements regarding limitations may include issues such as: the research approach, design, methods, sampling problems, uncontrolled variables, faulty administration of tests or training, generalizability of the data, representativeness of the subjects, compromises to internal and external validity, and issues related to the reliability and validity of the research instruments. The researcher should explain how he or she would control these limitations to accurately answer the research question.

9- Bibliography/References/Citations

These terms may be used interchangeably. In this section, the researcher should cite all citations that he or she has used throughout the proposal. Citations include all research articles, reviews, books and book chapters, monographs, etc. that a researcher refers to while writing the proposal. The references may be listed at the end of the proposal alphabetically or numbered according to the sequence that they appear in the text. Funding agencies usually provide guidelines as to how the references should be organized in the proposal.

C. ADMINISTRATIVE PLAN SECTION

In this section, the researcher explains how the proposal would be managed.

1- Time, Space and Availability of Equipment

The time required to complete the study should be anticipated. A timetable with specific tasks to be completed at specified times during the proposed study are always helpful and sometimes required by funding agencies. Resources available to the researcher to perform the study including, the instruments, laboratory space, computers, computer software, etc. should be explained in this section of the research proposal.

2- Budget

The requested budget should be discussed in detail as to how it will be spent (equipment, subject testing, subject reimbursement, salary of the investigator, travel, presentations at conferences, supplies, personnel, etc.).

3- Informed Consent Form

If the project involves the use of human subjects, the complete procedures for IRB approval of the project as well as procedures for acquiring the consent form and signatures from the subjects should be discussed.

SUMMARY

The research proposal is pivotal and necessary to any research study.

1. Without a proposal, research is at best unorganized and at worst useless.
2. The proposal is a powerful tool to help you learn, define, describe, and conduct useful research.
3. In writing a proposal, you must thoroughly research and accurately define your problem.
4. The research question you develop will define the appropriate experimental design.
5. Data management is essential for accurate conclusions.
6. Budgeting for your study is necessary to determine study needs, requirements, and feasibility for successful completion of your research project.

An Example of a Proposed Outline for Writing a Research Proposal

1- Long-term goals
2- Immediate purpose
3- Specific question(s) to be answered by this study
4- Research hypothesis (H_A)
5- Null hypothesis (H_o)
6- Operational definitions
7- Assumptions and limitations of the study
8- Types of study (descriptive, correlational, experimental)
9- Population
10- Sample
    a. Selection procedures
    b. Methods of selection and assignment
11- Independent variable(s)
12- Dependent variable(s)
13- Potential confounding variables and how they will be controlled
14- Research design
15- Level of measurement
16- Measurement tool(s)
17- Statistical tools (software packages, types of statistical tests)
18- Procedures (where is the data? how will it be obtained? how will it be used? Etc.)
19- Clinical application of the research
20- Anticipated problems
21- Informed consent
22- Time table
23- Budget
24- References

EXERCISES

1. In planning for research, do you first identify a problem area or try to find a testable hypothesis?
2. If you find conflicting results during your review of literature, in which part of the proposal will you discuss these issues?
3. If you use the review of literature to justify the importance of your research problem, which part of the proposal are you writing?
4. What is/are the differences between limitations and delimitations of the study?
5. A researcher is studying learning disabilities in children; however, he/she is only interested in children who are between the ages of 6-10 years old and who are living in low-income families. In which part of the proposal must he/she specify these requirements for her study?
6. In which section of the proposal should the researcher write his or her justification for the budget necessary to conduct the study?

QUESTIONS FOR DISCUSSION

1. Identify a problem area in your field and discuss three specific problems that could be investigated in that problem area.
2. If you have no idea about a research project, what is the most important first step of the process?

FOR STUDENTS DOING THEIR RESEARCH

Have you start writing your research proposal? If yes, what type of research design are you proposing, how many subjects, and what are the limitations and delimitations of your study?

NOTES

CHAPTER

19

RESEARCH COMMUNICATION

OVERALL OBJECTIVE

To become familiar with the procedural approaches to the various avenues available to present research results.

GOALS

1. Describe the format for research presented in a journal, at a conference or as a thesis
2. Illustrate the characteristics of a research report
3. Describe the sequence of events to be pursued in a presentation
4. Discuss the Do's and Don'ts of a presentation
5. Discuss how to critically review a research article

INTRODUCTION

The final and the most important stage of any research process is communication. Research would be of no value if the new knowledge acquired through the scientific process were not shared with others to improve the overall health of the society. The communication of research reports could be done as a published *article in a refereed journal*, as a *poster or oral presentation* in a scientific conference, or a *thesis* as part of a graduate student's work. The purpose of this chapter is to develop an understanding of these different processes and their characteristics.

General Characteristics of a Research Report

A research report in any format must be communicated with *clarity, organization, correct presentation, completeness, and conciseness.*

1. *Clarity:* The information must be communicated in a manner that is clear and easily understood.
2. *Organization:* The order in which the various parts of the report appear and the degree to which the transition between the parts are taking place must be comprehensible.
3. *Correct Presentation:* There should be a systematic format for the presentation of research material with proper spelling, grammar, dictation, and punctuation.
4. *Completeness*: The total body of facts should be presented to enhance clarity.
5. *Conciseness:* Any material that adds unnecessary length to the report must be eliminated.

FORMAT OF REPORTS

I. The Journal Article

There are several steps that a researcher must take before starting to prepare a manuscript for publication:

1- *Identifying a Journal for Submission.* First, the researcher must identify the appropriate journal in the related research field to which the manuscript will be submitted. Second, the researcher must review a few articles in each of the identified journals and examine the format used, as well as the required guidelines that must be followed for submitting an article to each journal. The selection of a journal must be based primarily on its orientation and type of readers. Most journals have specified the focus of their publication and the areas of interest to their readers. The researcher could evaluate and see which journal is more suited to publish the paper. Some papers may be rejected simply because the material is not in the same focus area of the journal and the readers. The focus of some journals is mainly research, some are practice oriented and are more appropriate for practitioners, some are highly specialized, and some are geared toward a general audience. Third, the researcher should try to find the manuscripts' acceptance rate of the journal; usually the acceptance rate is around 30% for very prestigious and specialized research journals, and 70% for practical general-audience journals.

2- *Submitting the Paper for Publication:* After identifying the appropriate journal, the researcher must carefully examine the requirements of the journal for publishing the manuscript including, presentation of material, illustrations, tables, and graphs. Each journal publishes the "Instructions for Authors" either on the journal or on their websites. The author must read that information and follow the instructions. An outstanding paper may be rejected if the authors do not follow the proper format or do not provide the information requested by the journal.

Components of a journal article

a. Abstract
b. Introduction
c. Methods
d. Results
e. Discussion
f. Tables and Graphs
g. Conclusions
h. References

a. Abstract. An abstract is usually the first thing seen in the manuscript, but is the last part that should be prepared by the author. It is the summary of the article in 150-200 words. The content of the abstract includes an overview of the study and its purpose, a brief description of methodology, the results, and a statement about the significance of the result and a conclusion.

b. Introduction. The introduction section is two to three paragraphs, which summarize the statement of purpose, background, and specific aims of the study and could be extracted from the same sections of the research proposal. Since the article is much shorter than a proposal, the researcher attempts (in two to three paragraphs) to state the importance of the study by stating the problem, providing some review of literature regarding the clinical relevance, rationale and theoretical framework of the study and follow up with a specific purpose and hypotheses (or guiding questions). After reading the introduction, the reader should have a clear understanding of the rationale behind the study, the question being asked, and the hypothesis being tested.

c. Methods. The methodology section should contain the study design, criteria for and methods of subject selection, description and number of subjects, measurement methods, data collection techniques, and data analysis procedures. This section could be taken directly from the research proposal. Note that the proposal is written in the future tense (you are proposing to do something in the future), the research article is written in the past tense since you are reporting what has been done. Nevertheless, it should be written in a much shorter length (page limitations) while clearly explaining the methodology utilized. All journals require that if human subjects were used for the research, they have been informed and the institutional review board of the institution approved the procedures. A statement of informed consent, procedures, and committees' approval must be included in this section.

d. Results. The results section of the manuscript should concisely state the statistical outcomes of the data. Author/s should not give any opinion at this time. The data is usually presented by depicting a narrative description of statistical outcomes, such as means and standard deviations of the demographics of the subjects (i.e., age, weight, height etc.). It will then continue by presenting the results of the statistical analysis and reporting the significance. Authors are encouraged to summarize their data in graphs and tables. Presenting tables of statistical analysis or graphing the results by identifying the significance might more clearly explain the data rather than trying to write everything down. The best way to logically report the data is for the author to go back to the objectives and hypothesis of the study and report the results accordingly.

Characteristics of Tables and Graphs

Tables and graphs are used to provide visual explanations of statistical findings and must follow guidelines for the specific journal. The most important characteristic of a table or a graph is that, both have to stand alone in representing the data, without the need for the reader to go back to the text to find out what they are representing. This means that if somebody without any knowledge of the content of the manuscript looks at the table or graph, he or she should be able to explain the results.

Components of a Table. Each table should have a title that specifically describes what is presented in the table, column headings (horizontally displayed) and a "field" within which the data is arranged by columns and rows. Sometimes the authors may include some footnotes to explain the characters that are summarized in the body of the table.

Example of a Table:

Table XX: Hypothetical Data on Physical Characteristics of Subjects

SUBJECT	SEX	Age (yrs)	WT (kg)	HT (cm)
1	M	32	96	182
2	F	40	40	149
3	M	38	106	190
4	M	31	105	182
5	M	30	67	188
6	M	26	67	188
7	M	40	56	167
8	F	37	52	162
9	M	56	110	182
10	M	48	84	188
11	M	20	86	182
12	M	24	60	180
13	M	34	72	170
14	F	34	51	172
AVERAGE		35	76	178
STD DEV		9.41	22	11.7

Components of a Graph. Graphs are usually used to more effectively depict the trends, relationships, and comparisons between the data. Data may be presented as a histogram, frequency polygon (line graph), pie chart, or bar graph.

Example of a Graph

Graph XX: Hypothetical Data on Percent change in heart rate during 30 minutes of exercise

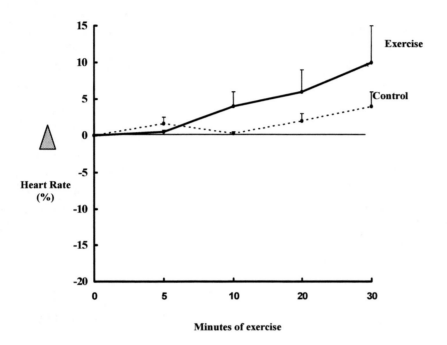

e. **Discussion.** The discussion section is the *focal point* of a research article. It reveals the interpretation of the results and is the only part where the researcher can express an opinion. It usually contains an interpretation of the statistical outcomes, clinical significance/importance of the work, comparison of the results with the work of others (using references), and how the results support or conflict with theory. The researcher may discuss the study's limitations and strengths and make suggestions for future research.

g. **Conclusion.** The conclusion is a brief summary of the purpose of the study and the study's principal findings. The author links the summary of the results and the meaning of those results with clinical implications and proposes future directions for the research.

h. **References.** In this section, the researcher should record all the citations that he or she has used throughout the article. Citations include all the research articles, reviews, books and book chapters, monographs, etc. that a researcher refers to while writing the manuscript. The references may be listed alphabetically or numbered according to the way they appear in the text. Journals provide guidelines as to how the references should be organized in the paper.

PRESENTATIONS

Research may be presented at national, international, or local conferences as either a poster presentation or a platform presentation. The purpose is to disseminate new knowledge in a timely fashion. The audience is usually limited to the members of that professional organization and the results will only be published as an abstract either in the proceedings of the conference or in a journal related to the conference. It may serve to obtain peer review/feedback before publication of the research as a full-refereed article.

Poster Presentation

A poster presentation is presenting the research results on a large board (usually 8 X 4 feet) so that it can be read and viewed by a group at once. Researchers are usually allocated a time and space at a conference to display their research and to informally discuss the findings with small groups (usually 5 to 8 people). A poster is usually made up of 10-15 matted panels that include a title banner (long, 5-6 feet), 1 panel for the abstract, 1 for the introduction, 2-3 for methodology, 2-4 for the results (including tables and graphs), 1 for the conclusion, and 1 for implications of the study and acknowledgments.

Abstract.
The abstract is usually less than 200 words and includes the problem, the purpose, methods used, a summary of important results, a conclusion, and the implications of the study.

Introduction.
This is one to two paragraphs, usually in bullet format that specifies the problem, needs, significance, objectives and hypotheses of the study.

Methodology.
The methodology section includes the design of the study, subjects, and procedures used including the data analysis techniques. Usually researchers use photos of equipment and set-up to depict the experimental procedures.

Results.
The results present the essential data. Usually color graphs and tables are used to depict the results.

Conclusions and Implications.
This section talks about the absolute bottom-line or take-home message(s) from the study! It is the "What do you want your audience to learn about your project? What does this study imply? What is the need for future studies?"

Acknowledgments. Researchers are encouraged to acknowledge the sponsors, funding grant agency, medical supervision, special assistance or moral support, consultant, specialist, or subjects of the study.

Example of a Poster

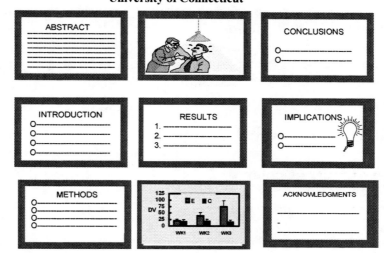

Do's of a Poster Presentation

1- Clarity and simplicity
2- Legible: should be able to read from 6 feet away
3- Bullets: Use key words
4- Title: 1.0-1.5" tall
5- Authors, etc.: 0.5" tall
6- Pay attention to using visuals (use color, contrast, photos, figures, tables)
7- Use the logos of your institution

Don'ts

1- Illegibility: using small fonts (< 18-pt font) that can not be read from 6 feet away
2- Long narratives
3- Too many numbers
4- Too many abbreviations
5- Too much information

6- All text; no figures
7- Typographical errors

Platform Presentation

These are usually 10 - 15 minute talks with 5-10 minutes for questions and discussion. The researcher has "one chance to make a good impression" and must say the most important points about the research in 10 to 15 minutes. Usually, it is presented in a linear sequence of 10-15, 35-mm slides or computer images (e.g., PowerPoint). The sequence and components of the images are like the poster presentation. The researcher must time himself or herself to be able to discuss all of the slides in a timely manner. Usually you should allow about 15 seconds for the title and introduction of yourself and your research group, 2 minutes for the introduction and rational of the study, 30 seconds for the purpose of the study, 3 minutes to discuss the methodology, 5 minutes to present the results, and 5 minutes for the discussion and conclusion. The final slide usually depicts the acknowledgments and opens the forum for questions and discussion.

Do's for a platform presentation

1- Answer questions politely
2- Admit mistakes
3- Welcome constructive criticism
4- Minimize speculation
5- Practice before the presentation and time yourself

Don'ts:

1- Illegibility (less than 18-point font)
2- Too many numbers, abbreviations, information, etc.
3- Rush, mumble, sound bored, or read from the slides

THESIS PREPARATION

A thesis is required as part of the graduation requirements for some masters degrees and all PhD degrees. Depending on the program and institution's requirements, the format of a thesis may be different. Nonetheless, it is usually arranged in three major parts.

Part I: Preliminary Items
Part II: Text
Part III: Supplementary Items

PART I: PRELIMINARY ITEMS

The preliminary items are usually included as separate pages at the beginning of a thesis and include the title page, acceptance page, acknowledgments, table of contents, list of tables, list of figures, and an abstract.

PART II: THE TEXT

The text or the body of a thesis is a comprehensive and detailed description of the entire study and usually consists of five chapters.

Chapter 1: Introduction. The introduction chapter usually includes the following sections: Introduction, Statement of the Problem, Purpose of the Study, Need for, Significance of, or Justification for the Study, Delimitations, Limitations, Assumptions, and Hypothesis. You will notice that this section is exactly the same as the sections in a research proposal. Therefore, the researcher can transfer this information from his or her already written research proposal to the thesis.

Chapter 2: Review of Literature. This section includes a review of the related literature and should be well organized and all citations must be recorded correctly. The review of literature must show how the present study is different from previous ones, how it is the same, and how it will contribute to the research area under investigation. Statements on how your study will fill in the knowledge gap based on the review of literature should be included.

Chapter 3: Methodology and the Procedures for Collecting Data. This section is presented as a systematic and careful plan for attacking the problem. The procedures for subject selection, methodology, and techniques that were used to conduct the study must be explained in detail with step-by-step instructions for conducting the study. The methodology section of the thesis should answer the following questions:

1- What variables were measured and how were they controlled?
2- How were the characteristics or variables measured?
3- What types of measuring system/equipment were utilized?
4- How many subjects were selected?
5- How were the subjects selected?
6- What types of sampling procedures were used?
7- Were the extraneous variables controlled?
8- Who collected the data and how?
9- How were the threats to internal and external validity controlled?
10-What was the timeline for the completion of the study?

Chapter 4: Data Analysis/Results. In the data analysis section, the emphasis is on reporting the results only. No opinion regarding the interpretation of the results should be made. This chapter should begin with an opening paragraph that restates the problem and tells the reader how the chapter is organized. For example, the following sections may be used:

1- Data gathering procedures
2- Demographic data
3- Statistical analyses techniques used
4- Presentation of the findings, using graphs and tables

The most important characteristic of this section is that the researcher must report the data in an unbiased manner and without expressing any opinion. Both the supporting and non-supporting data, with regards to the original question or hypothesis, must be presented.

Chapter 5: Discussion. This section is the most important part of a thesis. The author is expected to offer an educated and justified opinion regarding the interpretation of statistical outcomes. He or she should discuss the clinical significance of the outcomes, the importance of the work, and how the results support or conflict with theory. A comparison of the results with the work of others is encouraged. Author should, without any bias, discuss the limitations and strengths of the study and make suggestions for future studies.

Chapter 6: Summary/Conclusion/Implications. Any of the above titles may be used for this section. In this section, the author should state the problem, give a general overview of the source of data and the methods used and list the most important findings. Author should not make conclusions beyond the data obtained and should not over speculate. There should be some recommendations on how he or she envisions the findings being applied.

Chapter 7: References. The references may be alphabetized or numbered according to their appearance in the text.

PART III: SUPPLEMENTAL ITEMS/APPENDICES

Student may present some of the information as an appendix in the thesis, such as: documentation of materials and instruments, consent form, and protocol/instructions to the subjects.
In general, the thesis basically follows the same format as a research article, however it is much more extensive and should be presented in more detail.

SUMMARY

In summary, reporting the research is necessary to disseminate new knowledge. There are several avenues to report the results of research. Depending on your professional status and your research, you may decide which path to take. The most important point is that when reporting your research, the presentation must be accurate, concise, and interesting to your audience. As a researcher, you should always be proud of what you have accomplished and contributed to your discipline.

CRITICAL REVIEW OF A RESEARCH ARTICLE

Reading a research article and gaining new knowledge is one of our professional responsibilities; however, we have so little time and so many things to do in our every day lives. Therefore, the articles that we read should be presented in an effective and correct manner so that we may find it useful to incorporate it into our own practice or use it as a foundation to build more research. Hence, critical reviews of research articles are an important professional responsibility. The purpose of this section is to provide some practical approaches to the critical reading of published materials and to evaluate them for their accuracy and importance.

You may use this approach for your own research writing before submitting your paper for publication. It should be noted that, when you submit a manuscript to a refereed journal it goes through the same critical review by the experts in the field before it is accepted for publication. The following points should be considered when reviewing a research article:

1- **Introduction:** Every research article published should have a stated purpose. The reader should not have to search for the purpose or to identify the research question. If you cannot find the purpose of the study or the question asked in the introduction section of the paper, do not waste your time reading the rest of the paper. The research question is an important part of a research article. It dictates the design and methodology for data collection. For example, if the research question is a descriptive research question, the authors should not have an experimental design with dependent and independent variables. However, if the research question is correlational or experimental, there is always some component of descriptive research inherent in the data analysis. For example, the author may present the descriptive analysis of data just to show the overall characteristics of the subjects or use frequency distributions to see how the data looks. Overall, the *Pyramid of Research Knowledge* moves from descriptive to correlational to experimental or comparative.

PYRAMID OF RESEARCH KNOWLEDGE

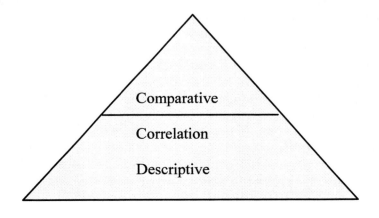

2- **Methodology:** This is a precise plan of action that an investigator follows to answer the research question. It should be written in a language precise enough to allow for duplication of the study.

3- **Results:** Statistical analysis for the interpretation of the data must be appropriate for the level of measurement used in the study. For example, parametric statistics should not be used to evaluate a set of nominal data. The result must be clear in answering the research questions and examining the research hypothesis. The characteristics of the tables and graphs should meet the requirements that were discussed earlier.

4- **Discussion:** Authors must be up-to-date on previous and ongoing research in their area. In the discussion section, attention should be made to use more recent literature and only discuss the research that is related to the results of the study. Authors should not over speculate their results or generalize to a population other than the one studied.

In general, when reviewing a research article, you should be able to answer the following questions:

1. Did the author answer the question that was asked?
2. Was the methodology appropriate and unbiased with strong internal validity?
3. Were the results unbiased?
4. Was the review of literature related to the results of the study and was it used to draw sound, logical conclusions?
5. Was the discussion/conclusion justified by evidence?
6. Are the results applicable to clinical situations?

EXERCISES

1- Why do we have to communicate the results of our research with others?
2- Can a researcher initiate the data collection process for his or her research and write the proposal for the study during his or her free time afterward? Why yes? Why no?
3- What is/are the difference (s) between a research proposal and a research article?
4- What is the "Guidelines for Authors" which is published in most journals?

5- If a researcher is in the middle of his or her study, but finds some very interesting results and wants to share it with others, should she/he present it as a research article or a conference presentation? Why?

6- What does the Pyramid of Research Knowledge mean, and how can it help us with a critical review of an article?

7- In which part of a research article should you be able to find the research question (s) and purpose of the study?

8- In which part of an article do the researchers discuss their subject selection criteria?

9- In which part of an article are the researchers allowed to express their opinions?

QUESTIONS FOR DISCUSSION

1- You read a research article and find that there are some major ethical problems with the study that have not been discussed in the article. What would you do?

2- How do you decide which research article is worth reading?

FOR STUDENTS DOING THEIR RESEARCH

1- If you are doing a thesis, have you started writing the preliminary sections of your thesis, including the introduction, review of literature, and methodology?

NOTES

APPENDIX I

ADDITIONAL READINGS

ADDITIONAL READINGS

1. American Evaluation Association (1994). *Guiding principles for evaluators*. New Directions for Evaluation, 66, 19-26.

2. American Psychological Association (1994) *Publication Manual of the American Psychological Association*, (4th edition). Washington, DC: American Psychological Association.

3. Black, T.R. (1999) *Doing Quantitative Research in the Social Sciences: An Integrated Approach to Research Design, Measurement and Statistics*. Thousand Oaks, CA: Sage Publications.

4. Bordens, K. S. & Abbott, B. B. (1996) *Research Design and Methods: A Process Approach* (3rd ed.) Mountain View: Mayfield.

5. Borenstein, M., & Cohen, J. (1988). *Statistical power analysis: A computer program*. Hillsdale, NJ: Erlbaum.

6. Borenstein, M., Cohen, J., Rothstein, H. R., Pollack, S., & Kane, J. M. (1995). *Statistical power analysis for one-way analysis of variance: A computer program. Behavior Research Methods, Instruments, & Computers, 22*, 271-282.

7. Campbell, D. T. & Stanley, J. C. (1963) *Experimental and Quasi-Experimental Designs for Research* Boston: Houghton Mifflin.

8. Carmines, E. and Zeller, R. (1979). *Reliability and Validity Assessment*. Newbury Park: Sage Publications.

9. Cohen J. (1988) *Statistical Power Analysis for the behavioral science*. 2nd ed. Hillsdale, NJ: Lawrence Erlbaum Associates.

10. Cone, J.D., & Foster, S.L. (1993) *Dissertations and theses from start to finish*. Washington, DC: American Psychological Association.

11. Converse, J. and Presser, S. (1986). *Survey Questions: Handcrafting the Standardized Questionnaire*. Newbury Park: Sage Publications.

12. Cook, T. D. & Campbell, D. T. (1979) *Quasi-Experimentation: Design & Analysis Issues for Field Settings* Boston: Houghton Mifflin.

13. Denzin, N.K., & Lincoln, Y.S. (Eds.) (1994) Handbook *of qualitative research*. Thousand Oaks, CA: Sage. Chapter 27. Huberman, A.M. & Miles, M.B. "Data Management and Analysis Methods".

14. Fowler, F.J. (1988) *Survey Research Methods*, Second Edition. Newbury Park: Sage Publications.

15. Gelfand, H., & Walker, C.J. (1990) *Mastering APA style: Students workbook and training guide*. Washington, DC: American Psychological Association.

16. Green SB, Salkind NJ, Akey TM. (1997) *Using SPSS for Windows: Analyzing and Understanding Data.* Upper Saddle River, NJ: Prentice-Hall.

17. Guba, E.G., & Lincoln, Y.S. (1989). *Fourth generation evaluation*. Newbury Park, CA: Sage.

18. Henderson, K.A. (1991) *Dimensions of Choice: A Qualitative Approach to Recreation, Parks & Leisure Research*. State College, PA: Venture Publishing.

19. Hinton, P. (1995) *Statistics Explained: A Guide for Social Science Students*. London: Routledge Publishing.

20. House, E.R. (1994) *Principled Evaluation: A critique of the AEA guiding principles*. New Directions for Evaluation, 66, 27-34.

21. Kantowitz et al. *Reliability and Replication: Analogical Reasoning...* pp343-352. In Experimental Psychology, 4th Edition (1991).

22. Kerlinger, F. N. (1994) *Foundations of Behavioral Research* (2nd Ed.) New York: Holt, Rinehart and Winston.

23. Krejcie, R.V.& Morgan, D. W. (1970) *Determining sample size for research activities. Educational and psychological measurements.* 30, 607-610.

24. Kim, J.O. and Mueller, C. (1978) *Factor Analysis: Statistical Methods and Practical Issues*. Newbury Park: Sage Publications.

25. Knapp TR. (1996) The Overemphasis on Power Analysis. Nurse Res. 45:379-80.

26. Middleton, M.R. (2000) *Data Analysis Using Microsoft Excel: Updated for Office 97 & 98.*

27. Nicol, A.A.M, & Pexman, P.M. (1999) *Presenting your findings: A practical guide for creating tables.* Washington, DC: American Psychological Association.

28. Rossi, P.H. (1994) *Doing good and getting it right. New Directions for Evaluation,* 66, 55-60.

29. Salant, P. and D. A. Dillman (1994). How to conduct your own survey. John Wiley & Sons, Inc.

30. Shaughnessy and Zechmeister (1994) *Quasi-Experimental Designs and Program Evaluation.*pp 325-360 in Research Methods in Psychology, 3rd Edition.

31. Trochim, W.M.K. (1989). *Introduction to concept mapping for planning and evaluation. Evaluation and Program Planning,* 12, 1-16.

32. Trochim, W. and Land, D. (1982). *Designing designs for research.* The *Researcher,* 1, 1, pgs. 1-6.

33. Wallgren, A., Wallgren, B., Person, R., Jorner, U., & Haaland, J. (1996) *Graphing Statistics and Data: Creating Better Charts.* Thousand Oaks, CA: Sage Publications.

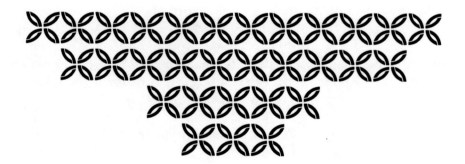

APPENDIX II

GLOSSARY OF STATISTICAL TERMS

GLOSSARY OF STATISTICAL TERMS

ABSCISSA: The horizontal or X-axis of the coordinate system. On a frequency distribution, the abscissa typically measures the variable in question (performance measures), whereas the Y-axis (ordinate represents the frequency of occurrence).

ALPHA ERROR (OR TYPE I ERROR): The probability of being wrong whenever the null hypothesis is rejected, or the probability of rejecting the null hypothesis when it should have been accepted. By definition, then, the alpha error can only occur when H_o has been rejected.

ALTERNATE HYPOTHESIS: The opposite of the null hypothesis. The alternate hypothesis states that chance has been ruled out--that there are population differences (when testing the hypothesis of difference), or that a correlation does exist in the population (when testing the hypothesis of association).

ANALYSIS OF VARIANCE: Statistical test of significance developed by Sir Ronald Fisher. It is also called the F ratio or ANOVA for Analysis of Variance. The test is designed to establish whether or not a significant (non-chance) difference exists among several sample means. Statistically, it is the ratio of the variance occurring between the sample means to the variance occurring within the sample groups. A large F ratio, occurs when the variance between is larger than the variance within and usually indicates a non-chance or significant difference.

BETA COEFFICIENT (B) OR SLOPE: In a scatter plot, the slope of the regression line indicates how much change on the Y variable accompanies a one-unit change in the X variable. When the slope is positive (lower left to upper right), Y will show an increase as X increases, whereas a negative slope (upper left to lower right) indicates a decrease in Y and is accompanying an increase in X. In the regression equation, $Y = bX + a$, the slope is symbolized by the b term.

BETA ERROR (OR TYPE II ERROR): The probability of being wrong whenever the null hypothesis is accepted, or the probability of accepting the null hypothesis when it should have been rejected.

BIAS: Sampling error, which is not random. Occurs when the difference between X and μ is consistently in one direction. Bias results when samples are not representative of the population.

CENTRAL LIMITS THEOREM: The theoretical statement that when sample means are selected randomly from a single population, the means will distribute normally, even if the population distribution deviates from normality. The theorem assumes that sample sizes are relatively large (at least 30) and that they are selected from one population.

CENTRAL TENDENCY (MEASURES OF): A statistical term used for describing the typical, middle, or central scores in a distribution of scores. Measures of central tendency are used when the researcher wants to describe a group as a whole with a view toward characterizing that group on the basis of its most common measurement. The researcher wishes to know what score best represents a group of differing scores. The three measures of central tendency are the mean (or arithmetic average), the median (or the midpoint of the distribution), and the mode (the most frequently occurring score in the distribution).

CHI SQUARE (X^2): A statistical test of significance used to determine whether or not frequency differences have occurred on the basis of chance. Chi-square requires that the data be in nominal form, or the actual number of cases (frequency of occurrence) that fall into two or more discrete categories. It is considered to be a non-parametric test (no population assumptions are required for its use). The basic equation is as follows:

$X^2 = \sum (f_o - f_e)^2 / f_e$

Where f_o denotes the frequencies actually observed and f_e the frequencies expected on the basis of chance.

COEFFICIENT OF CONTINGENCY (C): A test of correlation on nominal data sorted into any number of independent cells.

COEFFICIENT OF DETERMINATION (R^2): A method for determining what proportion of the information about Y is contained in X; found by squaring the Pearson r.

COEFFICIENT OF VARIATION: The coefficient of variation measures the spread of a set of data as a proportion of its mean. It is often expressed as a percentage. It is the ratio of the sample standard deviation to the sample mean.

CONFIDENCE INTERVAL: The range of predicated values within which one can expect with a certain degree of certainty that the true parameter value will fall. Usually, confidence intervals are determined on the basis of a probability value of .95 (95% certainty) or .99 (99% certainty).

CONFIDENCE LIMITS: Confidence limits are the lower and upper boundaries/values of a confidence interval, that is, the values which define the range of a confidence interval.
The upper and lower bounds of a 95% confidence interval are the 95% confidence limits. These limits may be taken for other confidence levels, for example, 90% or 99%.

CONTROL GROUP: In experimental research, the control group is the comparison group, or the group that receives zero magnitude of the independent variable. The use of a control group is critical in evaluating the pure effects of the independent variables on the measured responses of the subjects.

CORRELATED *F* RATIO: Statistical test of the hypothesis of difference among several sample means, where sample selection is correlated. The correlated *F* requires interval data.

CORRELATED SAMPLES: In experimental research, two or more samples that are not selected independently. The selection of one sample determines how the other sample(s) will be selected, as in a matched-group design.

CORRELATED T RATIO: Statistical test of the hypothesis of differences between two sample means, where the sample selection is correlated. The correlated *t* requires interval data.

CORRELATION COEFFICIENT: A quantitative formulation of the relationship existing among two or more variables. A correlation is said to be positive when high scores on one variable associate with high scores on another variable, and low scores on the first variable associate with low scores on the second. A correlation is said to be negative when high scores on the first variable associate with low scores on the second, and vice versa. Correlation coefficients range in value from +1.00 to –1.00. Correlation coefficients falling near the zero point indicate no consistent relationship among the measured variables. In social research the correlation coefficient is usually based on taking several response measures of one group of subjects.

CRITICAL REGION: The critical region of the sampling distribution of a statistic is also known as the alpha region. It is the area, or areas, of the sampling distribution of a statistic that will lead to the rejection of the hypothesis tested when the hypothesis is true.

 CRITICAL VALUE: The critical value or values of a statistic is the value(s) of that statistic that cut off the proportion of the sampling distribution designated as the alpha region(s).

CRAMER'S V: A test of correlation on nominal data when the number of independent cells is greater than four.

CROSS-SECTIONAL RESEARCH: Type of non-experimental research, sometimes used to obtain data on possible growth trends in a population. The researcher selects a sample (cross section) at one age level, say 20-year-olds, and compares these measurements with those taken on a sample of older subjects, say 65-year-olds. Comparisons of this type are often misleading (today's 20-year-olds may have very different environmental backgrounds, educational experiences, for example, than the 65-year-old subjects have).

DECILES: Divisions of a distribution representing tenths, the first decile representing the 10th percentile, and so on. The 5th decile, therefore, equals the 50th percentile, the 2nd quartile, and the median.

DEGREES OF FREEDOM (DF): With interval (or ratio) data, degrees of freedom refer to the number of scores free to vary after certain restrictions have been placed on the data. With six scores and a restriction that the sum of these scores must equal a specified value, then five of these scores are free to take on any value whereas the sixth score is fixed (not free to vary). In inferential statistics, the larger the size of the sample, the larger the number of degrees of freedom.
With nominal data, degrees of freedom depend, not on the size of the sample, but on the number of categories in which the observations are allocated. Degrees of freedom are based on the number of frequency values free to vary after the sum of frequencies from all of the cells has been fixed.

DEPENDENT VARIABLE: In any antecedent-consequent relationship, the consequent variable is called the dependent variable. The dependent variable is a measure of the output side of the input-output relationship. In experimental research, the dependent variable is the effect half of the cause-and-effect relationship, whereas in correlational research the dependent variable is the measure being predicted. In the social sciences, the dependent variable is typically a response measure.

DESCRIPTIVE STATISTICS: Techniques for describing and summarizing data in an abbreviated, symbolic form; shorthand symbol for describing large amounts of data.

DEVIATION SCORE (X): The difference between a single score and the mean of the distribution. It is found by subtracting the mean, X, from the score X. The deviation score (x - x) is symbolized as x. Thus $x = (x - x)$.

DISTRIBUTION: The arrangement of measured scores in order of magnitude. Listing scores in distribution form allows the researcher to notice general trends more readily than with an unordered set of raw scores. A frequency distribution is a listing of each score achieved, together with the number of individuals receiving that score. When graphing frequency distributions, one usually indicates the scores on the horizontal axis (abscissa) and the frequency of occurrence on the vertical axis (ordinate).

DOUBLE-BLIND STUDY: A method used by researchers to eliminate experimental error. In a double blind study neither the individual conducting the study nor the subjects are aware of which group is the experimental group and which is the control. This prevents any unconscious bias on the part of the experimenter, or any contaminating motivational sets on the part of the subjects.

EXCLUSION AREA: The extreme areas under the normal curve. Because of the curve's symmetry, the extreme areas at both the top and bottom of the curve are excluded by two z scores, which are equidistant from the mean.

EXPERIMENTAL DESIGN: Techniques used in experimental research for creating equivalent groups of subjects. There are three basic experimental designs: 1) after-only--where subjects are randomly assigned to control and experimental groups and the dependent variable is measured only after the introduction of the independent variable; 2) before-after--where a group of subjects is used as its own control, and the dependent variable is measured both before and after the introduction of the independent variable; 3) matched-group--where subjects are matched or equated, person for person, on some relevant variable.

EXPERIMENTAL RESEARCH: Research conducted using the experimental method, where an independent variable is manipulated (stimulus) in order to bring about a change in the dependent variable (response). Using this method the researcher is allowed to make cause-and-effect inferences. Experimental research requires careful controls in order to establish the pure effects of the independent variable. Equivalent groups of subjects are formed, then exposed to different stimulus conditions, and then measured to see if differences can be observed.

FACTORIAL ANOVA: As opposed to a one-way ANOVA, the factorial ANOVA allows for the analysis of data when more than one independent variable is involved. Results can be analyzed on the basis of the effects of each independent variable or on the basis of the possible interaction among the independent variables. Data to be analyzed should be at least interval form.

FISHER, SIR RONALD (1890-1962): English mathematician and statistician who developed the analysis of variance technique, or F (for Fischer) ratio.

FREQUENCY POLYGON: A graphic display of data where single points are plotted above the measures of performance. The height where the point is placed indicates the frequency of occurrence. The points are connected by a series of straight lines.

FRIEDMAN ANOVA BY RANKS (X_R^2): A test of the hypothesis of difference on ordinal data when the sample groups have either been matched or a single sample has been repeatedly measured. The Friedman ANOVA is the ordinal counterpart of the correlated F.

GALTON, SIR FRANCIS (1822-1911): The "father of intelligence testing" and the creator of the concept of individual differences, Galton, introduced the concepts of regression and correlation (although it was left to his friend and colleague Karl Pearson to work out the mathematical equations).

GAMBLER'S FALLACY: An erroneous assumption that independent events are somehow related. If a coin is flipped ten times and comes up heads each of those times, the gambler's fallacy predicts that it is virtually certain for the coin to come up tails on the next flip. Since each coin flip is independent of the preceding one, the probability remains the same (.50) for each and every coin flip, regardless of what has happened in the past. The gambler remembers the past, but the coin does not.

GAUSS, KARL FRIEDRICH (1777-1855): German mathematician credited with having originated the normal curve. For this reason the normal curve is often called the Gaussian curve.

GOSSETT, WILLIAM SEALY (1876-1937): Using the pen name "Student", Gossett, while working for the Guinness Brewing Company in Ireland, developed the technique of using sample data to predict population parameters, which led to the development of the *t*- test.

HALO EFFECT: A research error arising from the fact that people who are viewed positively on one trait are often also thought to have many other positive traits. Advertisers depend on this effect when they use famous personalities to endorse various products--anyone who can throw touchdown passes *must be* an expert in evaluating razor blades. Researchers must guard against the halo effect, as it will contaminate the independent variable.

HAWTHORNE EFFECT: A major research error due to response differences resulting not from the action of the independent variable, but from the flattery or attention paid to subjects by the experimenter. Typically, the potential for this error is inherent in any study using the before-after experimental design without an adequate control group. Any research, for example, where subjects are measured, then subjected to some form of training, then measured again, should be viewed with suspicion unless an appropriate control group is used--that is, an equivalent group that is measured, then not subjected to the training, and then measured again. Only then can the researcher be reasonably confident that the response differences are due purely to the effects of the independent variable.

HISTOGRAM (BAR GRAPH): A graphic representation of data in which a series of rectangles (bars) are drawn above the measure of performance. The height of each bar indicates the frequency of occurrence.

HOMOGENEITY OF VARIANCE: An assumption of both the *t* and *F* ratios, which demands that the variability within each of the sample groups being compared should be fairly similar.

HOMOSCEDASTICITY: The fact that the standard deviations of the Y score along the regression line should be fairly equal. Otherwise the standard error of estimate is not a valid index of accuracy.

INCLUSION AREA: The middlemost area of the normal curve, including the area between two z scores equidistant from the mean. Because of the symmetry of the normal curve, the middlemost area includes, in equal proportions, the area immediately to the left of the mean and the area immediately to the right of the mean.

INDEPENDENT VARIABLE: In any antecedent-consequent relationship, the antecedent variable is called the independent variable. Independent variables may be manipulated or assigned. A manipulated independent variable occurs when the researcher deliberately alters the environmental conditions to which subjects are being subjected. An assigned independent variable occurs when the researcher categorizes subjects on the basis of some preexisting trait.
Whether the independent variable is manipulated or assigned determines whether the research is experimental (manipulated independent variable) or *post-facto* (assigned independent variable). In experimental research, the independent variable is the causal half of the cause-and-effect relationship. In correlational research, the independent variable is the measure from which the prediction will be made.

INDUCTIVE FALLACY: An error in logic resulting from over-generalizing on the basis of too few observations. The inductive fallacy occurs when one assumes that all members of a certain class have a certain characteristic because one member of that class has it. It would be fallacious to assume that all Mongolians are liars on the basis of having met one Mongolian who was a liar.

INFERENTIAL (PREDICTIVE) STATISTICS: Techniques for using the measurements taken on samples to predict the characteristics of a population-- the use of descriptive statistics for inferring parameters.

INTERDECILE RANGE: Those scores that include the middlemost 80% of the distribution, or the difference between the 1st and 9th quartiles.

INTERQUARTILE RANGE: Those scores that include the middlemost 50% of the distribution, or the differences between the 1st and 3rd quartiles.

INTERVAL DATA: Data (measurements) in which values are assigned such that both the order of the numbers and the intervals between the numbers is known. Thus, interval data not only provides information regarding greater-than or less-than status, but also information as to how much greater or less than.

KRUSKAL-WALLIS *H* TEST: A test of the hypothesis of difference on ordinal data among at least three indecently selected random samples. The H test is the ordinal counterpart of the one-way ANOVA.

KURTOSIS (KU): The state or degree of the curvature of a unimodal frequency distribution. Kurtosis refers to the peakedness or flatness of the curve.

LEPTOKURTIC DISTRIBUTION: A unimodal frequency distribution in which the curve is relatively peaked--most of the scores occur in the middle of the distribution--with very few scores occurring in the tails. A leptokurtic distribution yields a relatively small standard deviation.

LONGITUDINAL RESEARCH: A type of *post-facto* research in which subjects are measured repeatedly throughout their lives in order to obtain data on possible trends in growth and development. An example of this research technique is Terman's* massive study of growth trends among intellectually gifted children. The study, begun in the early 1920s, is still in progress today and is still providing science with new data. Longitudinal research requires great patience on the part of the investigator, but the obtained data is considered to be more valid than that obtained using the cross-sectional approach.
*Terman LM. *Genetic Studies of Genius.* Stanford, CA: Stanford University Press; 1925, 1926, 1930, 1947, 1959.

MANN-WHITNEY U TEST: A test on ordinal data of hypothesis of difference between two independently selected random samples. The *U* test is the ordinal counterpart of the independent *t* test.

MCNEMAR TEST: Technique developed by the statistician Quine McNemar that uses chi-square for the analysis of nominal data from correlated samples.

MEAN (X): A measure of central tendency specifying the arithmetic average. Scores are added and then divided by the number of cases. The mean is best used when the distribution of scores is balanced and unimodal. In a normal distribution, the mean coincides with the median and the mode. When the entire population of scores is used, the mean is designated by the Greek letter (mu).

MEASUREMENT: A method of quantifying observations by assigning numbers to them on the basis of specific rules. The rules chosen determine which scale of measurement is being used: nominal, ordinal, interval, or ratio.

MEDIAN (MDN): A measure of central tendency that specifies the middlemost score in an ordered set of scores. The median always represents the 50th percentile. It is the most valid measure of central tendency whenever the distribution is skewed.

MESOKURTIC: A unimodal frequency distribution whose curve is normal (see Normal Curve).

MODE (MO): A measure of central tendency that specifies the most frequently occurring score in the distribution of scores. When there are two most-common points, the distribution is said to be bimodal.

MULTIPLE R: *A* single numerical value that quantifies the correlation among three or more variables.

MULTIPLE REGRESSION: Technique using the multiple R for making predictions of one variable given measures on two or more others. It requires the calculation of the intercept (a) and also at least two slopes (b_1 and b_2). For the three-variable situation, the multiple regression equation is as follows: $Y = a + b_1X + b_2X^2 + b_3X^3$

NOMINAL DATA: Data (measurements) in which numbers are used to label discrete, mutually exclusive categories; nest counting data, which focuses on the frequency of occurrence within independent categories.

NON-PARAMETRIC: Statistical tests that neither predict the population parameter, μ, nor make any assumptions regarding the normality of the underlying population distribution. These tests may be run on ordinal or nominal data, and typically have less power than parametric tests.

NORMAL CURVE: A frequency distribution curve resulting when scores are plotted on the horizontal axis (X) and frequency of occurrences is plotted on the vertical axis (Y). The normal curve is a theoretical curve shaped like a bell and fulfilling the following conditions: 1) most of the scores cluster around the center, and as we move away from the center in either direction there are fewer and fewer scores; 2) the scores fall into symmetrical shape--each half of the curve is a mirror image of the other; 3) the mean, the median, and mode all fall at precisely the same point, the center; and 4) there are constant area characteristics regarding the standard deviation.

NULL HYPOTHESIS: The assumption that the results are simply due to chance. When testing the hypothesis of difference, the null hypothesis states that no real differences exist in the population from which the samples were drawn. When testing the hypothesis of association, the null hypothesis states that the correlation in the population is equal to zero (does not exist).

ODDS: The chances against a specific event occurring. When the odds are 5 to 1, for example, it means that the event will not occur five times for each single time that it will occur.

ORDINAL DATA: Rank-ordered data, that is, ordinal measures that provide information regarding greater-than or less-than status, but not how much greater or less.

ORDINATE: The vertical Y-axis in the coordinate system. As a frequency distribution, the ordinate indicates a frequency of occurrence.

PARAMETER: Any measure obtained by having measured the entire population. Parameters are, therefore, usually inferred rather than directly measured.

PARTIAL CORRELATION: Correlation technique that allows for the ruling out of possible effects of one or more variables of the relationship among the remaining variables. In a three-variable situation, the partial correlation rules out the influence of the third variable on the correlation between the remaining two variables.

PASCAL, BLAISE (1623-1662): French mathematician and philosopher who introduced the concepts of probability and random events.

PEARSON, KARL (1857-1936): English mathematician and colleague of Sir Francis Galton. It was Pearson who translated Galton's ideas on correlation into precise mathematical terms, creating the equation for the product-moment correlation coefficient, or the Pearson r.

PEARSON r: *Statistical* technique introduced by Karl Pearson for showing the degree of relationship between two variables. Also called the product-moment correlation coefficient, it is used to test the hypothesis of association, that is, whether or not there is a relationship between two sets of measurements. The Pearson r can be calculated as follows:

$$r = n \sum xy - (\sum x)(\sum y) / \sqrt{([n \sum x^2 - (\sum x)^2][n \sum y2 - (\sum y)^2])}$$

Computed correlation values range from +1.00 (perfect positive correlation) through zero to -1.00 (perfect negative correlation). The farther the Pearson r is from zero, whether in a positive or negative direction, the stronger is the relationship between the two variables. The Pearson r can be used for making better-than-chance predictions, but cannot be used for isolating causal factors.

PERCENTILES: The percentage of cases falling below a given score. Thus, if an individual scores at the 95th percentile that individual has exceeded 95 percent of all persons taking that particular test. If test scores are normally distributed, and if the standard deviation of the distribution is known, percentile scores can easily be converted to the resulting z scores.

PERCENTILE RANK: The value that indicates a given percentile. A person at the 75th percentile is said to have a percentage rank of 75.

PHI COEFFICIENT: A test of correlation on nominal data when a number of independent cells are exactly 4 (that is 2×2 chi square analysis).

PLATYKURTIC DISTRIBUTION: A unimodal frequency distribution in which the curve is relatively flat. Large numbers of scores appear in both tails of the distribution. A platykurtic distribution of scores yields a relatively large standard deviation.

POINT OF INTERCEPT (a): In a scatter plot, the point of intercept is the location where the regression line crosses the ordinate, or the value of Y when X is equal to zero. In the regression equation, $Y = bX + a$, the intercept is symbolized by the a term.

POPULATION: The entire number of persons, things or events (observations) having at least one trait in common. Populations may be limited (finite) or unlimited (infinite).

POST-FACTO RESEARCH: A type of research that, while not allowing for cause-and-effect conclusions, does allow the researcher to make better-than-chance predictions. In such research, subjects are measured on one response dimension and these measurements are compared with different response measures. Responses are compared with responses, as in comparing the SAT scores with grade-point averages for a group of students. Since the experimenter does not treat the subjects differently (there is no manipulation of an independent variable), cause-and-effect conclusions may not be drawn from *post-facto* data.

POWER (1 – β): A measure of the sensitivity of a statistical test. The more powerful a test is, the less is the likelihood of committing the beta error (accepting the null hypothesis when it should have been rejected). The higher a test's power, the higher the probability of a small difference or a small correlation being found to be significant.

PROBABILITY (P): A statement as to the number of times a specific event/s, can occur out of the total possible number of events. Probability should be expressed in decimal form. Thus, a probability of 1 out of 20 is written as .05.

QUARTILES: Divisions of a distribution representing quarters; the 1st quartile representing the 25th percentile, the 2nd quartile the 50th percentile (or median) and the 3rd quartile the 75th percentile.

QUOTA SAMPLING: Selecting a sample directly reflects the population characteristics. If it is known that 45% of the population is composed of males, and if it is assumed that gender is a relevant research variable then the sample must contain 45% of male subjects.

RANDOM SAMPLE: Samples selected in such a way that every element or individual in the entire population has an equal chance of being chosen. When samples are selected randomly, then sampling error should also be random and samples should be representative of the population.

RANGE (R): A measure of variability that describes the entire width of the distribution. The range is the difference between the two most extreme scores in a distribution, and is, thus, equal to the highest value minus the lowest value.

RATIO DATA: Data (measurements) that provide information regarding the order of numbers, the difference between numbers, and also an absolute zero point. It permits comparisons, such as A being three times B, or one-half B.

REGRESSION LINE: The single straight line that lies closest to all of the points in a scatter plot. The regression line can be used for making correlational predictions when three important pieces of information are known: 1) how much the scatter points deviate from the line, 2) the slope of the line, and 3) the point of intercept ($Y = bX + a$).

REPRESENTATIVE SAMPLE: A sample that reflects the characteristics of the entire population. Random sampling is assumed to result in representative samples.

SAMPLE: A group of any number of observations selected from a population, as long as it is less than the total population.

SAMPLING DISTRIBUTIONS: Distributions made up of measures taken on successive random samples. Such measures are called statistics, and when all samples in an entire population are measured, the resulting sampling distributions are expected to be normal (See Central Limits Theorem). Two important sampling distributions are the distribution of means and the distribution of differences.

SAMPLING ERROR: The expected difference between the mean of the sample and the mean of the population ($x-\mu$). Under conditions of random sampling, the probability of obtaining a sample mean greater than the population mean is identical to the probability of obtaining a sample mean less than the population mean (P = .50).

SCATTER PLOT: A graphic format in which each point represents a pair of scores, the score on X as well as the score on Y. The array of points in a scatter plot typically forms an elliptical shape (a result of the central tendency usually present in both the X and Y distributions).

SECULAR TREND ANALYSIS: A method using the regression technique to predict trends across time. Historical data are used for predicting future results, based on the assumption that the past trend will continue.

SIGNIFICANCE: A statistical term used to indicate that the results of a study are not simply a matter of chance. Researchers talk about significant differences and significant correlations, the assumption being that chance has been ruled out (on a probability basis) as the explanation for these phenomena.

SKEWED DISTRIBUTION: An unbalanced distribution in which there are a few extreme scores in one direction. In a skewed distribution, the best measure of central tendency is the median.

SPEARMAN, CHARLES E. (1863-1945): English psychologist and test expert who worked in the area of measuring intelligence and identifying factors that make up intelligence. In pursuing his correlational studies on intellectual factors, he produced a correlation technique for the analysis of ordinal data called the Spearman rho, or r.

SPEARMAN R: Correlation coefficient devised by Charles E. Spearman for use with rank-ordered (ordinal) data. Sometimes called the Spearman ρ (rho).

STANDARD DEVIATION (SD): A measure of variability that indicates how far all scores in a distribution vary from the mean. The standard deviation has a constant relationship with the area under the normal curve (see Normal Curve).

STANDARD ERROR OF DIFFERENCE: An estimate of the standard deviation of the error distribution of differences between pairs of successively and randomly selected sample means. The estimate can be made on the basis of the information contained in just two samples.

STANDARD ERROR OF ESTIMATE (Se_{est}): A technique for establishing the accuracy of a predicted Y value obtained by using the regression equation. The higher the correlation between r and Y, the lower the resulting value of the standard error of estimate and the more accurate the predicted Y value is. When $r = 0$, the standard error of estimate is equal to the standard deviation of the Y distribution.

STANDARD ERROR OF MEAN (S_X): An estimate of the standard deviation of the entire distribution of random sample means successively selected from a single population until that population has been exhausted. This estimate can be made on the basis of information contained in a single sample, that is, the standard deviation of the sample and the size of the sample.

STATISTIC: Any measure that is obtained from a sample as opposed to the entire population. The range (or the standard deviation or the mean) of a set of sample scores is a statistic.

SUM OF SQUARES (SS): An important concept for ANOVA; the sum of squares equals the sum of the squared deviation of all scores around the mean. When the sum of squares is divided by its appropriate degrees of freedom, the resulting value is called the mean square, or variance.

***T* RATIO:** Statistical test used to establish whether or not a significant (non-chance) difference exists between two sample means. It is a ratio of the difference between two sample means to an estimate of the standard deviation of the distribution differences.

T SCORE: A converted standard score such that the mean equals 50 and the standard deviation equals 10. The scores, thus, range from a low of 20 to a high of 80.

TUKEY'S HSD (HONESTLY SIGNIFICANT DIFFERENCE): A technique developed by J.W. Tukey for establishing whether or not the differences among various sample means are significant. The test is performed after an ANOVA only when the F ratio is significant.

UNIMODAL DISTRIBUTION: A distribution of scores in which only one mode (most frequently occurring score) is present.

VARIABILITY MEASURES: Measures that give information regarding individual differences, or how persons or events vary in their measured scores. The three most important measures of variability are range, standard deviation, and variance (which is the standard deviation squared).

VARIABLE: Anything that varies and can be measured. In experimental research, the two most important variables to be identified are the independent variable and the dependent variable. The independent variable is a stimulus, is actively manipulated by the experimenter, and is the causal half of the cause-and-effect relationship. The dependent variable is a measure of the subject's response and is the effect half of the cause-and-effect relationship.

VARIANCE: A measure of variability that indicates how far each of the scores in a distribution vary from the mean. Variance is equal to the square of the standard deviation.

WILCOXON T TEST: A test on ordinal data of the hypothesis of difference between two sample groups when the selections are correlated (as in the matched-group design). The Wilcoxon T is the ordinal counterpart of the correlated t.

YATES CORRECTION: A correction factor applied to a 2 x 2 chi square analysis (or anytime $df = 1$) whenever any of the expected frequencies are less than 10. The difference between f_o and f_e is reduced by .50 resulting in a slightly lower chi square value.

Z SCORE (STANDARD SCORE): A number that is the result of the translation of a raw score into units of standard deviation. The score specifies how far above or below the mean a given score is in standard deviation units. A score above the mean converts to a positive z score while scores below the mean convert to negative scores. The z score is also referred to as a standard score. The mean of the z score distribution is equal to zero.

APPENDIX II

TABLES OF RANDOM NUMBERS AND SAMPLE SIZE